HEALTH at the Crossroads

Exploring the Conflict Between Natural Healing and Conventional Medicine

Dean Black, Ph.D.

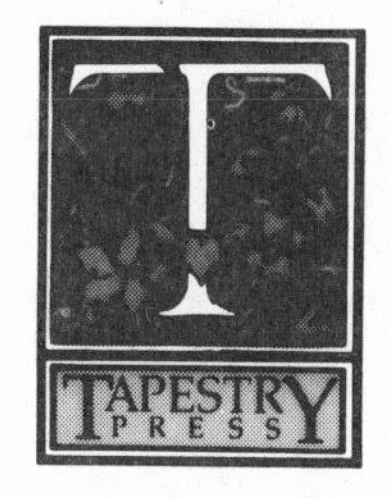

PO Box 653, Springville, UT 84663 (801)489-9432

The information in this book is presented as a matter of general interest only and not as prescribing cures or recommending treatments. Readers must use their own judgment, and consult a natural healing expert or their personal physician for specific applications to their individual needs. Although the author and publisher have made every effort to ensure the accuracy and completeness of information contained in this book, we assume no responsibility for errors, inaccuracies, omissions, or any inconsistency herein. Any slights of people or organizations are unintentional.

Library of Congress Cataloging-in-Publication Data

Black, Dean, 1942-
Health at the Crossroads : exploring the conflict between natural healing and conventional medicine / Dean Black
p. cm.
Bibliography: p.
Includes index.
ISBN 0-929283-17-1 : $9.95. ISBN 0-929283-07-04 (pbk.) : $5.95
1. Medicine—Philosophy. 2. Alternative medicine—Philosophy.
3. Health. I. Title
R723.B56 1988
610'.1—dc19 88-21994
CIP

ATTENTION HEALTH PROFESSIONALS, COLLEGES AND UNIVERSITIES, GOVERNMENT AGENCIES:
Quantity discounts are available on bulk purchases of this book for patient, educational, or promotional use. For information, please contact our Special Sales Department, Tapestry Press, P.O. Box 653, Springville, UT 84663.

Printed and bound in the United States of America.

For Claudia, Laurie, Brent, David, Melissa, Adam, Kimberli, Christopher, Jennifer, Triana, Michael, and Philip, who are my family.

ACKNOWLEDGMENTS

I gratefully acknowledge Dr. Tei-Fu Chen, whose patient explanations of the Chinese healing philosophy first provoked my interest in this topic. I received valuable comments and suggestions on the content of the book from Fuller Royal, Randy Wysong, Loren Israelsen, Clinton Miller, Catherine Frompovich, Judith Todero, Burton Kallman, Steven Foster, Joe Pizzorno, Paul Lee, and Robert Arbon. I thank Tom and Marilyn Ross for their perceptive editorial assistance, and for helping me discover the name of the book. And for support that was neither editorial nor academic, but invaluable nonetheless, I thank Robert Lovell, Marv Peterson, Rae Howard, Don Stevens, and many, many others who shared hope and encouragement along the way.

Contents

Introduction

An 84-year-old man had cancer. Chemotherapy wasn't working for him, so his doctors turned to what they called "BCG immunotherapy." Unfortunately, the therapy, which involves injecting the patient with bacteria, caused an infection, and the patient died from it. But when the doctors did an autopsy, they found his tumors had shrunk, which pleased them. In fact, they published a report of his case in which they wrote that, though the patient died of "disseminated BCG infection . . . the arrested growth of his tumors is best attributed to the beneficial effect of BCG immunotherapy."

I was intrigued when I read this, then pleased a bit myself — not that the patient died, but to have been given such a clear example of my thesis, which is this:

Medicine is a way of thinking. Being logical and consistent, it produces predictable outcomes, some of which aren't good, and have put medicine in a state of crisis. I'm referring here to medicine's loss of public esteem, the twin challenges of treatment-caused illness and malpractice suits, and the persistence of chronic illnesses like cancer, arthritis, and heart disease. Medical thinking can't overcome the crisis, because the problems that cause it come straight from medical logic. Good intentions won't help, nor will hard work, until we back them with a healing logic that produces the outcomes we seek. That healing logic will balance medicine with a gentler principle.

In the case of the 84-year-old man, medical logic gave the doctors two separate goals. One was to save the patient; the other was to defeat the cancer. At first glance, they seem like the same goal, but the logic of medicine assures they are not. By the logic of medicine, the disease is separate from the patient. It is an "entity," to use the proper word, which my dictionary defines as "something that exists independently and apart from other things." Saving the patient is one goal. Defeating the separate and independent entity called cancer is another.

To use a World War II analogy, the patient's body is like a French village that's been invaded by German soldiers, who are the cancer. The doctors are U.S. soldiers who've been called in to defend the village, a duty that charges them with two responsibilities: (a) to beat the Germans, and (b) to save the village. Of the two, beating the Germans represents the higher cause. If you have to destroy the village to do it, that's one of the risks of war.

Medicine wages war against cancer, not simply as one person's suffering, but as a scourge against humankind. That war transcends any individual. When the 84-year-old patient's doctors spoke of the "beneficial effects" of the therapy that killed him, they spoke abstractly of the progress of the war, or more aptly, of the outcome of a real-time weapons test. Perhaps in another battle, defending another village, we might not only reduce the tumor, but (if we can just avoid the fatal infection) save the patient as well.

There is, of course, a certain logic to this. Nevertheless, it also produces an impersonal objectivity in the doctor-patient relationship, the same objectivity that must guide a general who sends soldiers into battle, knowing as he does that villages will burn and soldiers will die. This objectivity has nothing to do with a general's or a doctor's personal emotions; it may even cause them anguish of soul. Impersonality is simply a requirement of leadership in all military professions, of which medicine is but one, though differing from other military professions in the nature of its enemies and the battlegrounds on which its battles are fought.

By separating the disease from the patient and casting the doctor opposite the disease in a military posture, medicine's logic fixes the doctor's attention on the disease, not on the patient. This almost guarantees that patients will find doctors distant and cold. Not that doctors can't create deeply personal moments with their patients; many of them do. But to do this, they literally exchange their medical frame of mind for another. Medical logic, by itself, is inherently cold and impersonal, and so are doctors when they assume the role it creates for them.

(When I use the word "doctor," by the way, I refer, not to individual practicing physicians, but to a mythical, prototypical physician who faithfully and faultlessly acts out the logic of classical medicine, untempered by any other principle. My mythical doctor is also male, since I've settled on the generic masculine pronoun as the simplest, most readable solution to the fact that English has no genderless pronouns.)

Medical thinking also produces a certain therapeutic coarseness. Just as U.S. soldiers entered the French village as outsiders, doctors enter the body as outsiders. They *intervene* and *control*, essentially sticking thoughts and fingers into physiological processes that normally operate at the infinitely finer scale of our genes. By medical logic, they have to do this. It's their job, even though it requires that they impose a gross scale upon a finer one. Unfortunately, from time to time this virtually guarantees a bit of therapeutic heavy-handedness. We experience this as side-effects and treatment-caused illnesses such as the one that killed the 84-year-old cancer patient.

From such fabric, medicine fashions its own crisis.

In this book I suggest that medicine will never solve its crisis by working harder at the logic that created it. Instead we need a new healing logic that defines disease, not as the doctor's challenge, but as the patient's. Here the therapist's job isn't to wage war, but to encourage the patient's natural defenses. From this point of view, there can be no cause greater than the individual patient, because the patient *is* the cause. This healing principle exalts and supports the patient's natural adaptive powers.

The logic of natural healing produces its own predictable outcomes. For example, by not separating the patient from the disease, the logic of natural healing transforms therapeutic moments into personal moments. To talk about the disease is to talk about the patient. Patients like this warm and personal way of thinking.

The logic of natural healing also avoids medicine's coarseness. You can't heal the body by intervening and controlling; you've got to leave its inner processes alone. Let them do whatever they will at their own imperceptible scale. We'll find ways to support them that don't involve controlling them, or intruding our gross scale upon their finer one. From this sort of thinking, natural healing tends to produce neither side effects nor treatment-caused illnesses.

Whether or not it actually produces healing remains a separate question. Many people claim it does, giving as evidence the testimony of their own experience. I count myself among them. I had hay fever, and food allergies so severe they almost killed me. Cortisone helped, but I didn't like the side effects. Then I tried a natural healing remedy, and both the hay fever and the food allergies went away, without side effects. I'm pleased to be healed. And I believe the natural healing remedy did it, or at least helped my body do it.

The very gentleness that pleases patients and tends to avoid side effects also produces a certain conceptual and practical fuzziness that makes *proving* that natural healing did it almost impossible, at least to the satisfaction of classically trained scientists. As a result, those scientists generally call natural healing "unproven" and "unscientific," while it is actually neither. It is simply another way of thinking, as logical and internally consistent as medicine, and with its own methods of proof.

The logic of natural healing, however, also leaves an opening for charlatans. Unlike medicine, it places little value on explaining how a therapy works, so it doesn't concern itself with theory. Intending not to meddle, natural healing hardly ever considers what actually goes on inside the body. As a result, it doesn't depend nearly so much as medicine on having scientifically trained practitioners. In fact, much of natural healing is scarcely more complex than common sense — the sort of deep and richly informed common sense that most often comes from the accumulated experience of many lifetimes.

And natural healing is much more diverse than medicine. Anything that can affect the body's adaptive powers — which is virtually everything — may become part of natural healing, either recommended because it strengthens, or counselled against because it weakens. So natural healing, as a discipline, tends to be much more loosely defined than medicine, and hardly concise enough to allow such things as discipline-wide licensing boards of the sort that govern medicine. Besides, that sort of rigid external control doesn't fit well within a way of thinking based on the principle that bodies, and people, ought to be trusted to manage themselves.

So charlatans who choose health as their scam are much more likely to venture into natural healing than medicine, although medicine manages to produce a few charlatans of its own. And they find little to prevent them, other than the laws against economic fraud and — the best prevention of all — the educated discernment of the people they seek to cheat. In fact, the natural healing principle views charlatans much as it views germs: since it's almost impossible to destroy them, let's help people strengthen their defenses against them.

For reasons that lie beyond the scope of this book, certain segments of medicine have determined to do away with natural healing. They give the presence of a few charlatans as their excuse, though I suspect the matter is hardly that simple. These people wish to pass legislation that would outlaw natural healing, and give licensed medical doctors and licensed dieticians an exclusive claim to the health-care market.

This push to outlaw natural healing comes at a time when many people find themselves discontented with the coolness, coarseness, and cost of medicine, and turn for answers to the natural healing principle. The result is a conflict that becomes surprisingly heated and divisive for a profession whose goal is the sort of peace and wholeness that healing brings.

I hope in this book to clarify that conflict for nonscientists who are confused by it, and perhaps draw people from both sides of the conflict more peaceably together. I've tried to use non-technical language, and for the most part, I believe I've succeeded, largely because the logic involved is little more than simple common sense. However, chapters 3 and 5 ("Medicine Confronts the Second Law" and "Two Briefs in the Case Against Cancer") are a bit more technical. I believe you'll find them intriguing and worth the effort to understand. However, if you find yourself getting bogged down and wish to skip one or the other, you won't lose the thread of logic if you'll just read the last few transition paragraphs that lead to the next chapters.

Although the issues that define the conflict between natural healing and medicine are largely scientific and philosophical, they are also practical. We must choose therapists and therapies when we get sick. We're asked to vote on health-related laws and for the people who write them. These practical choices probably mean more than science or philosophy in setting the path that health-care will take in the future. If I do nothing more than help people make these choices more wisely and help preserve our freedom to make them, I will have achieved my goal.

1

Beware the Whoops! Factor

I once read a report about 12 joggers who had been attacked by buzzards while running through the birds' territory during their mating season. The report concluded with this advice: "Nature has its own laws and may not allow intrusion without revenge."

I got that same advice, more or less, from a man who owns a coffee plantation in Guatemala. I'd been driving with my family up a winding dirt road when a rock punctured our oil pan. A few moments later, the plantation owner happened by and offered to put us up for the night.

The next morning we toured his plantation. Germans built it, he explained, then abandoned it during World War II. He'd been rebuilding it over the past two or three years, hiring local Indians as labor. The local Indians were quite primitive, he said, and he'd tried to educate them. "I thought I could upgrade their standard of living," he explained, "but I gave up."

"Why?" I asked.

"Well," he said, "first I started an evening class in agriculture. About thirty Indians came. Then one day only one of them showed up — a man named Miguel. The next time even Miguel stayed home. I found out later that one of the other Indians had been visiting Miguel's wife while he was in class. Pretty soon everybody knew it but Miguel, so they all stayed home to protect their wives. Then Miguel figured out what was going on, and he stayed home, too. So I abandoned the class.

"Then I built an outhouse and encouraged the workers to use it. But they just squatted on the floor. I tried to teach them how to sit on the holes, but sitting just seemed to shut off their bowels. After a week or two of little piles on the floor, I tore the outhouse down."

Cultures, it appears, also have their own laws, and may not allow intrusion without revenge.

Here are other examples of the same principle:

- The moldboard plow with its long, straight furrows gave us the best-producing farms in the world. Now it appears it may have nearly destroyed those farms by letting the soil erode too fast.
- Officials of a midwest city's Department of Social Services set up Alcoholic Detoxification Centers to rehabilitate drunks at the cost of $86 per drunk per day. These centers replaced less well-equipped centers that cost only $9 per drunk per day. The centers ended up *increasing* the number of drunks, because being in the centers is more pleasant than being on the streets, and you can't get in them when you're sober.
- Most cities and towns set aside landfills for trash. Now experts estimate that landfills throughout the world put between 30 million and 70 million tons of methane gas into the atmosphere each year, making them a major threat to our atmosphere and climate.
- Laws designed to strengthen minority businesses exempted them from competitive bidding on certain "set-aside" government contracts. Reports now conclude that minority businesses have been weakened by the laws, and have a hard time weaning themselves from the set-aside programs and competing for traditional federal contracts.

I call this sort of thing the "Whoops! Factor," and I refer specifically to those cases where nature surprises us with outcomes we hadn't planned for. The Whoops! Factor goes beyond simple risk, where we enter an activity *know-*

ing there's a chance of failing, such as when we play the slot machines or have children. I'm speaking instead of those moments of naïve innocence when we honestly believe we've figured things out, only to end up worse off than when we started. When we least expect it, the Whoops! Factor transforms our noblest intentions into their opposite.

The Whoops! Factor in Medicine

Nowhere is this principle more common than in medicine. Take, for example, the "war on cancer." Congress declared war on cancer in 1971 when it passed the National Cancer Act. Since then, we've spent more than $25 billion on cancer research.

In 1985, a prominent cancer researcher named Robert T. Schimke made a startling admission about our progress in that war. Chemotherapy, he declared, tends to make cancer worse. The problem, he explained, is that cancer cells *resist* chemotherapy, and that resistance mimics the very processes of cancer itself. Dr. Schimke drew his conclusion from research sponsored by the American Cancer Society. He reported it in a lecture he gave at the National Institutes of Health in Bethesda, Maryland, where he was being honored for receiving the Alfred P. Sloan, Jr. Prize for his research. *Chemotherapy tends to make cancer worse*, this esteemed scientist said. This is serious Whoops! Factor territory.

No less sobering is what antibiotics do to bacteria. Scientists began searching for antibiotics during the late 1800's after Louis Pasteur formulated the germ theory of disease, and Robert Koch developed ways to isolate and identify varieties of bacteria. Today we've got more than sixty different antibiotics, all designed to kill bacteria.

But they also make the bacteria stronger. Today we face bacteria that didn't exist in Pasteur's and Koch's day, ones that even our best antibiotics won't touch. These bacteria have come to *resist* antibiotics. One study showed that, when an antibiotic was added to chicken feed, virtually all of the chicken's bacteria developed resistance to it within one week. Within six months, 80 percent of the farm family's bacteria were resistant as well, just from having been exposed to the chicken feed. Antibiotics also tend to weaken the immune system, rendering it more vulnerable to such stronger bacteria. Once again, our noblest intentions have been transformed into their opposite.

Curiously, both cancer cells and bacteria become stronger through the same physiological mechanism. It's called "gene amplification," and it means these enemies of ours actually *change their genes*. We don't like them, so we attack them. If they survive round one, they prepare for round two by altering themselves at the most fundamental level — the level of their genes.

Seeking an Alliance with Nature

The answer to these surprising Whoops! Factor outcomes would seem to be science. In a scientific sense, "surprise" and "information" are the same thing. The more something surprises us, the more it informs us. By the same token, the more informed we become, the less chance we have of being surprised. God, for example, being omniscient, cannot be surprised. Nor can he get a joke, since he knows all the punch lines. Likewise, when we know all there is to know about something, we eliminate surprising outcomes, since surprising outcomes are nothing more than punch lines to jokes we play on ourselves. And this is the Golden Promise of science. Every scientific discovery strikes some Whoops! Factor from our future. When science has discovered everything, we will have eliminated the Whoops! Factor altogether. Perhaps the ultimate scientific formula is this: perfect knowledge = perfect control. And this is its corollary: perfect control = no surprises.

This hopeful notion has established *control* as a key scientific concept. A poor scientific experiment is "uncontrolled." Conversely, a good experiment sets all of the proper "controls" firmly in place. And notice how these quotes link science with the promise of control:

- The philosopher Martin Heidigger saw in science a "will to dominate," leading it to become "a way of questioning things by which they are reduced to enslavement."
- Nobel prize winner Ilya Prigogine, speaking of

classical science, says, "The man of science now becomes a kind of magician . . . endowed with a potentially omnipotent knowledge."

- MIT biologist Robert A. Weinberg foresees a time when scientists will become able to "create versions of life that were never anticipated by natural evolution."

Our protection from the sort of power these quotes describe is the noble intentions that guide science. If the intentions that guide science manage to express themselves in the end, we shall have eliminated illness, ignorance, poverty, and war.

Yet if Whoops! Factor experiences have one message, it is this: intentions are not at the root of things, because they are too easily transformed into their opposite. There is some higher principle that must first be honored.

What I propose is that the buzzards have shown us that principle. *Nature has its own laws and may not allow intrusion without revenge*. Intrusion creates *resistance*, and it is resistance that transforms our noblest intentions into their opposite. The things we seek for ourselves — health, wisdom, prosperity, and peace — are all expressions of freedom, and freedom is the one thing we can't achieve through the principle of control. And if control can't give us freedom, neither can it give us anything else.

If that's true, our only choice is to seek a way of getting along with nature that doesn't pit us against her, that instead allies us with her, capturing her strength for our own. Does such a way exist? I believe it does. Our great challenge, in health and every other arena of life, is to find it.

2

Medicine Takes Healing From Nature's Hands

Medicine became scientific roughly the same time America became a nation. While our founding fathers debated politics, our medical fathers debated science. The questions the two groups debated were surprisingly similar. Our founding fathers asked, "Can a politically free people exist?" Our medical fathers asked, "Can a physiologically free body exist?" Our founding fathers answered, "Yes," to their question, and America was born. Our medical fathers answered, "No," to their question, and modern medicine was born.

The medical question, to be precise, was this: Does the body have innate adaptive powers that are sufficient to protect it from disease? America's most famous colonial doctor, Benjamin Rush (who also signed the Declaration of Independence), answered that question, in essence, as follows: "although a certain self-acting power does exist in the organism, it is subject to ordinary physical and chemical laws, and in any case, it is not strong enough to withstand the onslaughts of disease."

Having answered that question, Rush moved to a

second question that follows naturally from the first: given the body's apparent incapacity to defend itself, what shall the role of the physician be? To this Rush answered, "Although physicians are in speculation the servants, yet in practice they are the *masters of nature* . . . Instead of waiting for the slow operations of nature to eliminate a supposed morbid matter from the body, art *should take the business out of her hands*." (Italics added)

The "business," of course, is healing.

From that time to the present, medicine has developed as the science of taking the business of healing out of nature's hands. Medical therapies literally substitute for the healing power of the body. Antibiotics kill bacteria *in place of the body*. Chemotherapy kills cancer *in place of the body*. Drugs like insulin and cortisone regulate our chemical levels *in place of the body*. The new gene-splicing techniques promise even to determine our genetic potential *in place of the body*. As Benjamin Rush put it, although doctors may acknowledge the body's healing power *in speculation*, in practice scientific medicine's most fundamental premise directs them to become nature's masters.

Medicine's Two Basic Theories

In those Colonial days, Benjamin Rush and his colleagues sought to master nature by bleeding their patients and dosing them with a compound of mercury and chlorine called "calomel." Nowadays we've progressed to a much more sophisticated medicine based mainly on two theories about the causes and cures of disease: (1) the germ theory, and (2) the chemical imbalance theory.

According to the germ theory, diseases are caused by microorganisms that invade us and disturb our inner chemistry. Examples of the germ theory are the search for a way to kill the AIDS virus, and the recent concern over the reemergence of the tuberculosis bacillus. The medical goal here is to kill the germs before they kill us.

According to the chemical imbalance theory, we become sick when our body makes either too much or too little of certain active chemicals. Since these active chemicals control our body functions, having too much or too little of them makes our body functions too strong or too weak. Examples of the "chemical imbalance theory" are using insulin to manage diabetes, or anti-histamines to manage hay fever. Insulin *mimics* a body chemical, while anti-histamines *block* a body chemical. The medical goal in this case is to use either mimicking drugs or blocking drugs to bring the body's chemical levels back to normal.

Bitter Fruits of Medicine's Logic

Whether medicine succeeds or fails depends on the strength of these two theories. They are not the only theories of disease, simply the two that medicine has chosen. In many ways, medicine is not succeeding as well as doctors would like. For example, for all their successes, doctors must also contend with the fact that many people become sick from either medical errors or reactions to medical treatment.

Technically, illnesses caused by medical treatment are *iatrogenic*, which comes from two Greek roots: *iatros*, meaning physician, and *gen*, meaning origin, or source. Iatrogenic illness is illness whose source is the physician.

Iatrogenic illnesses are of two sorts: preventable and non-preventable. Preventable iatrogenic illnesses are medical mistakes or accidents. People who administer drugs sometimes give more or less than they should. Surgeons may nick arteries, or remove wrong organs. Patients get phlebitis from particles in the solutions that drip into their veins, or catch infections from other patients.

Non-preventable iatrogenic illnesses are side-effects of treatment that happen even to careful doctors. Here the treatment actually *causes* the illness, not because it's been wrongly done, but because it's inherently harmful. Doctors consider these the "risks" of modern medicine

If you look up iatrogenic illness in medical literature, here's some of what you'll find:

- Of all infants 60-days-old or younger who are hospitalized with fevers, twenty percent end up harmed by their medical treatment. Fourteen percent suffer from diagnostic errors. Twelve percent of the complications happen to infants who didn't need to be hospitalized.

- When researchers followed 3181 children who visited a general pediatric group practice during the course of one year, they found that more than 10% of them experienced one or more adverse drug reactions.
- In 25% of the cases where doctors use a particular diagnostic test, the test leads to entirely wrong results with severe therapeutic consequences.
- Six percent of patients who undergo a particular surgical implantation procedure develop colon cancer at the site of the implantation.
- The *New England Journal of Medicine* reports that 36% of 815 consecutive patients on a general medical service of a university hospital had an iatrogenic illness, and in 2% of the 815 patients, the iatrogenic illness was believed to contribute to the death of the patient.
- The *Journal of the American Medical Association* reports that 2.5% of patients admitted to an intensive care unit died from iatrogenic illness.

I called the Centers for Disease Control and asked how many patients die from iatrogenic illness each year. The researcher didn't know, so I presented these figures and asked her to help me figure it out. She found the number of hospital patients, and multiplying that by the 2% figure mentioned in the *New England Journal of Medicine*, we came up with 700,000 deaths. That 2% figure came from one study done at one hospital, and hospitals vary widely in their mortality rates, so it may not be accurate. A study published in 1974 put the figure at 0.5%, for example, which would put annual deaths from iatrogenic illness at about 175,000. I later found the 700,000 figure cited in another source, so perhaps it's not too far off. At any rate, the number is alarmingly high. AIDS killed roughly 30,000 people between 1981 and 1987. If my figures are correct, the number of direct and indirect deaths from iatrogenic illness during the same seven-year period falls somewhere between 1,000,000 and 4,000,000.

These deaths are as much a product of medicine's logic as are its successes. Scientifically, theories are only as good as their results. Are medicine's basic theories giving us the results we want? If not, why not?

The Germ Theory Overlooks the True Cause of Disease

The germ theory says that microorganisms cause infectious diseases like the scarlet fever, chicken pox, and the flu. Consider this, however: Let's say you and I sit talking with a friend who's got the flu. The flu virus finds its way from the friend into both of us, but only *I* get the flu; you don't. When that sort of thing happens — and it does all the time — the virus simply *cannot* be the cause. Something we have in common can't cause something we differ on, even though the virus is so connected to the flu that we can't get sick without it.

The basic logic of experimental science confirms this.

In a properly controlled experiment, you do what is called "matching your groups." You take the people you're going to do your experiment on, and divide them in half, like children choosing up teams on a playground. One team becomes your *experimental* group; the other team becomes your *control* group.

Since you want to find out what happens to people when you do something to them, you do it to your experimental group, but you *don't* do it to your control group. You create a difference, in other words, and you notice what other differences show up as a result. But if the groups *already* differ, you can't do this, or at least you get awfully confused. So you have to "match your groups." You make them as close to identical as possible, because whatever the two groups have in common you automatically eliminate as a possible explanation for whatever differences show up later.

In a major flu epidemic, it's almost impossible not to get exposed to the virus. And among those who get exposed, we end up with two groups: those who get flu and those who don't. To find out what caused the flu, we have to look at how the two groups differ, because what they have in common (including the virus) we automatically eliminate as a possible cause.

Here's a common-sense illustration of the point. Say I'm sitting on a bus reading the paper. I run across an article about a 35-car pileup on a Los Angeles freeway, turn to my seatmate and say, "Those freeways are *terrible*," as if the freeway caused the accident. The freeway, in this instance, is like the virus: you can't have a 35-car pileup without one. But the freeway is hardly the cause. To find the cause — something we can call *responsible* — we've got to find something that the problem *responds* to, something that's linked to the problem in such a way that, when *it* goes up and down, the problem goes up and down. In the case of freeway pile-ups, that's probably traffic density (I'm obviously oversimplifying here), since the denser the traffic, the more cars are likely to crash before traffic can adjust. We might even call the idea "scientific," in the sense that it's regular and lawful. As traffic density goes up at freeway speeds, so does the number of cars involved in the average accident.

Killing viruses to avoid the flu is more or less like tearing out freeways to avoid multi-car accidents. Yes, we could possibly do it. And, yes, we would eliminate one of the necessary conditions. But wouldn't it make more sense to work on the *responsible* variable, the one the problem *responds* to? In the case of multi-car accidents, we set as our goal to reduce traffic density. We stagger work hours, create incentives for businesses to move to the suburbs, or whatever. As traffic density goes down, so does the number of multi-car accidents, because we have addressed the cause.

In the case of the flu, the *responsible* variable is the weakness or strength of the body's adaptive powers. When our adaptive powers are weak, we're far more likely to get the flu. So we work on strengthening our adaptive powers, and as our adaptive strength goes up, our chances of getting the flu go down.

In both of these examples, we give our scientists a question to consider. For freeway scientists, the question is, "How can we reduce traffic density to prevent multi-car accidents?" For medical scientists, the question is, "How can we strengthen the body's adaptive powers to prevent the flu?" Both are legitimate and intriguing scientific questions.

But medical science, thanks to the way it's defined the germ theory, doesn't ask how to strengthen the body's adaptive powers. It asks how to kill germs. That's normally the body's job, of course, but medicine, as its central premise, takes that business for its own. The germs become stronger for being assaulted, while our adaptive powers become weaker for being replaced. At the very least, medicine's version of the germ theory is incomplete.

The Chemical Imbalance Theory Creates an Illusion

Does the chemical imbalance theory fare any better? By that theory, diabetes is an insulin deficiency, while hay fever is a histamine overload. We remedy the insulin deficiency by adding insulin from the outside; we remedy the histamine overload by neutralizing, or blocking, the histamine from the outside. But when we intrude with drugs in that fashion, our body compensates by adjusting its own chemical levels to cancel the effect of the drug.

This is known as the "bi-phasic" (or two-phased) effect of drugs. Phase one is what the drug does to the body; phase two is how the body adapts to the drug. The phases tend to go in opposite directions: the drug pushes; the body pushes back.

The result of this two-phased effect is a temporary illusion. For example, athletes sometimes take anabolic steroids. Anabolic steroids mimic the male hormone testosterone, which helps the body build muscle protein. Athletes who take steroids reason that, if they get extra testosterone, they'll build muscles more quickly. As they build more muscles in response to the outside testosterone, however, their body adapts by making less of its own, and they can end up with withered testicles and less testosterone than a normal man. On the outside they become more manly; on the inside, more feminine.

For another example, consider what happens when we block a class of body chemicals called endorphins. Endorphins, as one of their effects, depress breathing, and doctors have noticed that Sudden Infant Death Syndrome (SIDS) babies have higher-than-normal endorphin levels. Some doctors suspect, therefore, that the high endorphin levels depress the babies' breathing, causing them to die.

The way to handle this from the "chemical-imbalance" point of view would be to identify SIDS-prone babies and block, or neutralize, their endorphins. Some doctors have actually proposed this. It makes sense. If a baby risks death because it has too many endorphins, and if you get rid of some of them with an endorphin-blocking drug, you make the baby safer, or so it would seem.

But scientists once gave mice an endorphin blocker and noticed this two-phased effect that we've been talking about. The mice's level of active endorphins, as expected, went down. But two weeks later their bodies, to compensate, were producing 150 percent more endorphins than normal. They had adapted. Now imagine the same thing happening to those SIDS babies. If they were endangered before from too-high endorphins, how safe are they now that we've raised their endorphin level still higher? And lest we think this happens only in mice, studies show the same thing happening in humans.

As you can see, this two-phased effect means that drugs tend to worsen whatever they're supposed to cure, which sets up a vicious cycle. This is how street drugs addict. Most street drugs mimic natural body chemicals that relieve pain and make us feel good. As the street drug floods us with good feelings, our body compensates by moving our body chemistry in a direction that opposes those good feelings and causes us to depend on the drug. When the drug wears off, we feel worse, and if we persist in seeing the drug as our answer to unhappiness, we develop a stronger and stronger need for it. Medicinal drugs addict by the same principle.

How Medicine Ends Up Fighting the Body

In both the germ theory and the chemical imbalance theory, the adaptive powers we call *Life* enter only as an afterthought, and then mainly because they adapt, or resist. And no wonder. They are the very "hands" of nature from which medical science wishes to wrest the business of healing. Should we be surprised that the body wrestles back? Even my four-year-old knows enough to resist those who would wrest from him what he considers his own.

This well-meaning wrestling match between medicine and the body has set in motion a paradox that I can best explain with an example. When doctors try to get drugs to the brain, the body blocks the drugs through a mechanism called the *blood-brain barrier*. The blood-brain barrier *protects* the brain. It's part of the body's resistance. Yet if doctors are to get drugs to the brain, they must overcome it. When researchers finally broke through the blood-brain barrier, it was announced as a major medical breakthrough. The body's defeat became medicine's victory.

Yet doctors don't seek the body's defeat. Just the opposite. They wish only *health* for the body. But they couple their noble intention with a resolution (which their medical theory demands) that says, "I will achieve the body's health by imposing my will upon it." They seem not to consider that the body may have a will of its own. In their prescribed role as nature's masters, doctors succeed by defeating the body's will, even though the health they seek might properly be described as the ability to resist such defeat.

Of course, the body *does* resist, and this resistance has become one of medicine's major problems, sometimes almost as much of a challenge as disease itself. For example, I mentioned earlier Robert T. Schimke's prize-winning research on how chemotherapy provokes resistance that tends to make cancer worse. A *Science News* magazine article on the same topic carried this subtitle: "Researchers are struggling to learn how cancer cells survive in the presence of lethal drugs. *The aim is to prevent resistance*" (italics added). The article also pointed out where the cancer cells get this annoying resistance: they "retain whatever it is that allows the normal cell to persist in the presence of a toxic drug." The resistance, in other words, is a normal physiological mechanism, the very mechanism by which our cells defend themselves, yet doctors must now prevent it if they wish to continue using chemotherapy.

The answer in such cases is often a second drug to battle the resistance provoked by the first. Researchers discovered a body chemical that breaks up blood clots and began giving it as a drug to heart attack patients. They found that many of the patients got new clots ("reocclusion," it's called) quicker than ever. The reason, researchers discovered, is that these patients' bodies had begun to resist the effect of the clot-busting drug by producing "markedly elevated" levels of the *inhibitor* to it.

Now the inhibitor was "tipping the balance in favor of [clot formation]," which was the original problem. To handle this new turn of events, the researchers determined that they must now "find ways *to inhibit the inhibitor*" (italics added).

There's no question this sort of resistance hugely complicates medicine. The drug creates its advertised benefits; resistance reverses them. We may mask resistance by upping the dose of the original drug, or by introducing a second one, and for a time — perhaps for a long time — we may manage a tenuous balance that keeps the benefits ahead of the resistance. But I believe we may question the *principle* involved. While no one may doubt that careful *short-term* medical intervention saves many lives, the most fundamental logic of science argues that we can neither heal chronic illnesses nor nurture vibrant, long-term health by the same means. To do so, we would have to do the impossible. We would have to defy nature's most basic law.

3

Medicine Confronts the Second Law

At least part of the body's resistance to drugs comes from the operation of the Second Law of Thermodynamics. This law says that natural processes in *closed* systems move from order to chaos. (Closed systems are ones that don't receive energy from the outside.) To reverse that — to transform chaos into order — we've got to *add* energy, and all systems end up consuming more energy than they produce.

Every now and then someone claims to have invented a perpetual motion machine. Scientists scoff because a perpetual motion machine would violate the Second Law of Thermodynamics. I suggest that medicine faces the same barrier, that the law that reverses our well-intentioned medical intrusions is the Second Law of Thermodynamics. If that's true, the hope of overcoming the body's resistance to drugs is as doomed as the myth of perpetual motion.

To see why, let's look at our genes and what they do.

Genes Create Us by Making Proteins

Genes are *protein-makers*, and as they make their proteins, *we* come to exist. What makes proteins useful is their bumpy surfaces. They have nooks and crannies that let them grab hold of other molecules. In chemical terms, this grabbing is known as *binding*. Proteins *bind* to molecules, and in their binding, they lay, so to speak, the bricks that make us. We are, in a very real sense, stuck-together proteins.

Some proteins are *structural*, meaning they give us shape and keep us from coming apart. For the most part, these are bound-together copies of the same protein molecule. By binding to copies of themselves, structural proteins form fibers, sheets, rods, and tubes. These are what we see when we look at ourselves in the mirror, or see a lover across a candle-lit dinner table. Strange that so much can be made of stuck-together proteins.

Other proteins are much more dynamic and active. They attract and bind, not copies of themselves, but other molecules, many of which aren't proteins at all. These dynamic and active proteins may be antibodies of the immune system that bind to invaders. Or the hemoglobin in blood that binds to oxygen. Or chemical signals like hormones and neurotransmitters that bind to "receptors" on the surface of other cells, and so let the parts of us talk to one another.

Perhaps the most intriguing of these dynamic proteins are *enzymes*. Enzymes not only bind to molecules, they *transform* them. An enzyme may grab a single molecule, for example, and slice it in two. Or it may grab a molecule and rearrange it into another molecule. Or it may grab two or more molecules and stick them together to form a more complex molecule.

All of our chemical processes are brokered in this fashion by enzymes. When the body needs a chemical reaction, it creates, through the genes, an enzyme to handle it.

Actually, the body's chemical reactions could happen without enzymes. Enzymes just make them happen a million or more times faster. Some enzymes can process as many as two-and-a-half-million chemical reactions in a minute. So far, scientists have identified about 2000 enzymes, each with a set of nooks and crannies suited for its own particular brand of high-speed molecule making.

Folding and Tucking Through the Second Law

All proteins, whether enzymes or otherwise, are made from tiny building-block molecules called *amino acids*. To form a protein molecule, our genes first hook amino acids together in a string, attaching the head of one amino acid to the tail of another. Then the string gets folded and tucked in upon itself, and with this folding and tucking we arrive at a point in our physiology where the Second Law of Thermodynamics comes into play.

This folding and tucking is perhaps the most critical step in the protein-making process. It rounds the amino-acid string into a globe-like molecule, and, in the process, gives it those bumpy nooks and crannies that are just the right size and shape for binding molecules. If the folding goes wrong, the protein ends up with the wrong nooks and crannies and doesn't work.

You'd think, therefore, that the body would carefully guide the folding to make sure it happens just right. As a matter of fact, the body doesn't guide it at all. The folding happens automatically, guided only by the process known as "entropy," which is nature's process of randomization.

Actually, entropy isn't so much a process as a measure of *disorder*. The higher the entropy, the greater the disorder. Disordering means that things lose their connectedness, which makes them random. Families in a crowded park are islands of order within an otherwise random assembly. A little boy gets lost; entropy has increased. Family members scatter to look for him, and *they* get lost; entropy has increased still further. Thick fog settles in, so thick that *everybody* gets lost. Entropy is total; chaos is at its peak.

This drift toward chaos — toward *entropy* — is what happens when things get left to themselves. I look into my closet and see a scientific principle at work. This is the principle called the *Second Law of Thermodynamics*, and it says that all physical processes tend *irreversibly* to move in one direction — from a state of higher order to a state of lower order.

This is why we see logs burning into ash, for example, but never ash *un*burning into logs. Or why air rushes *from* a balloon, but never *into* a balloon. Or why a boulder rolls downhill, but not uphill. And it's why strings of amino acids fold the way they do, rather than some other way. Though the forces involved may differ, the principle is always the same.

Driven by nothing more than this Second Law of Thermodynamics, the amino acids in the string attract one another, and the folding simply follows the attractions, lines them up, and settles them into the simplest, most comfortable position. In chemical terms, the amino-acid string folds itself into the shape that *reduces its "free energy" to the lowest possible level*, which is the same thing a boulder does when it bounces down a hill. A bouncing boulder and the folding of a protein involve different forces, but the same principle guides them. Both processes are just as natural, just as automatic, and they don't need anyone, or anything, to direct them.

The Cost of Opposing the Second Law

Nor *could* anyone direct them without a high energy cost. Imagine stopping a bouncing boulder halfway down a slope, and holding it there. You could do it, but not without a cost. You've trapped the boulder's energy, and to keep it there, you would have to exert a biochemical energy equal to the gravitational energy you've trapped.

The situation would be *unnatural* now, because the boulder's tendency would be otherwise. You could hold it only by *opposing* its natural tendency. This would *not* be a self-sustaining situation. There would be a certain order to it, and you might count yourself pleased with it. But it is *your* order. You created it; you are responsible for it. If you decide you don't want to maintain *your* order, it unravels the instant you give it up, and the boulder bounds down the hill to *its* order, which is a state of rest at the bottom. That state of rest is the state of lowest free energy, because there's no more energy to be released within the natural order of things. You could dig a deep hole, roll the boulder to the edge of it, and push it in. You would have released more free energy, but that, again, would have been *your order*, and, in that sense, unnatural. Every natural situation has a certain configuration that represents its state of rest, and that is where it tends to move.

This, to me, is the marvel of the body. It creates life with processes that lead to entropy, or disorder, which is the *opposite* of life. These entropy-making processes cost the body nothing. They simply *flow*, and it would cost the body a great deal to oppose them. Of course, the body can't rely on entropy-making processes alone, because all they can do by themselves is disorganize us. So the body *opposes* entropy at certain key points.

For example, osmosis is one of these naturally flowing, entropy-making processes. It shifts fluids here and there, or moves molecules through membranes from one compartment of the body to another. Behind osmosis lies the Second Law of Thermodynamics and its natural flow toward entropy. Osmosis costs the body nothing.

But suppose the body wants a molecule to go from point A to point B, and osmosis would take it elsewhere. For this the body uses a process called *active transport*. Active transport carries molecules upstream, so to speak, against the flows of osmosis. It *opposes* entropy, which is like rolling a boulder up a hill. Once active transport gets the molecule to point B, it releases it, and, like a boulder released at the top of a hill, the flow of osmosis naturally and easily takes it somewhere else.

The trick the body has mastered so well is knowing exactly which biochemical hilltops to carry things to so that life is created through naturally unfolding, entropy-driven processes, and the total energy expended when all is said and done is as low as possible. Virtually all of the body's biochemical processes *end* with these entropy-driven reactions, but they generally begin with reactions that oppose entropy, and must therefore be jump-started, so to speak, by drawing on energy from the body's energy stores, which come from the food we eat.

So we can divide the body's chemical reactions into two categories: (1) those that oppose entropy and must therefore be driven by energy drawn from the body's energy stores, and (2) those that are driven by the natural flow of entropy-making processes and cost the body nothing. Our point for this discussion is that the protein-folding that we talked about is driven, like osmosis, by the entropy-making processes of the Second Law of Thermodynamics.

How the Second Law Powers Enzymes

The Second Law of Thermodymanics not only folds amino acid strings into enzymes, it also guides and powers the enzyme in its work. I mentioned earlier that enzymes "broker" chemical reactions. They use their nooks and crannies to bind molecules in order to split them in two, or to combine simple molecules to form more complex ones. The critical thing about those nooks and crannies is that they allow the enzyme to arrange the molecules in a configuration that lets them *lose free energy*. Once they reach that configuration, that's what they do — lose free energy — naturally and spontaneously. As they lose free energy, they change. Losing free energy *transforms* them. Molecule A becomes Molecule B. Or Molecules A and B join to become Molecule C.

This is how enzymes make molecules like insulin, cortisone, and adrenalin. These molecules *do* things to the body. They are *active*, *powerful* chemicals. It is by making these active chemicals — or more accurately, by making the *enzymes* that make these active chemicals — that the genes govern our body chemistry. And at the heart of it all is the Second Law of Thermodynamics, in the form of entropy-driven processes that follow natural tendencies, and proceed, unguided, to the state of lowest free energy that *attracts* them as surely as gravity attracts a boulder.

How the Second Law Sets our Chemical Levels

Not only does the body use the Second Law of Thermodynamics to make active chemicals, it uses it again as it keeps the amounts of those active chemicals at critical, life-sustaining levels. Imagine an enzyme whose job is to transform Molecule A into Molecule B. Around the enzyme we place 10 molecules of Molecule A. The enzyme grabs one and transforms it into Molecule B. Now we have nine A molecules and one B molecule. The enzyme grabs another A, transforms it, and now we have eight A's and two B's. Notice that each transformation changes the *ratio* of A molecules to B molecules.

This is important because changing the ratio between the molecules also changes the free energy available in the situation, and there is a *particular ratio* where the free energy is as low as it can be. On either side of that ratio, the free energy rises, just as slopes rise on either side of a valley. This makes all other ratios unnatural for our body, just as it's unnatural for that bouncing boulder to stop for a rest on a steep slope.

Now, let's suppose that the ratio with the lowest free energy is four A molecules for every six B molecules. In that case, the enzyme will automatically and naturally transform A's to B's — or B's to A's — until it reaches that lowest-free-energy ratio — that is, until there are four A's for every six B's. At that ratio, the free energy is at its lowest, and, like the boulder settling into the valley, the transforming will stop.

The transforming is more or less like a pendulum. It can swing either of two ways, and always tends to settle at the lowest point. Too many A's push the transformation to one side; too many B's push it back. The *attraction*, in either case, is toward that valley in the middle.

How Medicine Opposes the Second Law

As medicine has developed, it has come more and more to explain health and disease in terms of the levels of those active chemicals that our enzymes make for us. The power of this point of view is that it immediately suggests logical therapies. When the cause is too little of a molecule (as in the case of diabetes), we therapeutically *add* it from the outside. When the cause is too much of a molecule (as in the case of hay fever with its histamine overload), we therapeutically *block* it from the outside. As we discussed in the last chapter, this is what drugs typically do. They add to our supply of an active chemical, or they block it. In this fashion, the doctor adjusts our molecule levels up or down, depending on what he perceives to be the problem.

Now, consider what goes on in the body. Even though the doctor doesn't like the molecule levels the body has chosen for itself, they are nonetheless the ones the body has chosen. And it has chosen them in a very simple way: it has allowed them to follow their natural tendency to settle in the valley of lowest free energy. When the doctor arbitrarily changes those levels, he simply shifts them to a state of higher free energy, which is like pushing a boulder halfway up a hill. The new molecule levels are *not* the body's order. They are the doctor's order. He has chosen them; he must sustain them. Yet as often as he pushes the molecule levels uphill, they simply settle again into the valley of lowest free energy, and thus oppose the direction the doctor wishes to push them. They have no choice. That is the body's design and nature's law.

Medicine's Findings Undermine Its Own Basic Principle

Two-hundred years ago, Dr. Benjamin Rush declared, in essence, "Although a certain self-acting power does exist in the organism, it is subject to ordinary physical and chemical laws, and in any case, it is not strong enough to withstand the onslaughts of disease." Physicians, therefore, "are the masters of nature," and should "take the business [of healing] out of nature's hands." Modern medicine, from that time until now, has been constructed on that basic principle.

Medicine's dilemma is that its own findings undermine its basic principle. If the body's self-acting power is "subject to ordinary physical and chemical laws," medicine has yet to find them, as witnessed by the ease with which the body resists chemotherapy and other drugs. If the body's self-acting power is "not strong enough to withstand the onslaughts of disease," medicine has found nothing stronger, as witnessed by the ease with which bacteria resist antibiotics.

Believing in the supremacy of the body's adaptive powers is no longer "unscientific," as shown by this quote from *The Skeptical Inquirer*, a journal published by Carl Sagan:

> Modern science has taught us that the human body, insofar as it is cured, tends to cure itself. The body is its own greatest protector: the immunological system, which produces antibodies to fight antigens, accounts for almost all recovery from disease . . . *Nothing can save the patient if the internal system breaks down* . . . This is not to belittle medicine; its

> discoveries are prodigious and its contributions to health salutary, but the success of modern medicine depends on an understanding *of how the healthy body protects itself.* (Italics added.)

More than a few medical doctors now sense the truth of those thoughts and accept the shift in thinking they imply. By seeking to understand how the healthy body protects itself, they are beginning to add to their medical principles an equally valid set of natural healing principles — those that account for the body's *natural* adaptive powers.

Yet the transition to natural healing is far from complete. Most medical doctors still hold tenaciously to the old idea of external control. Shifting to the new principle won't be easy. One complication is the fact that the natural healing principle is the very one that scientific medicine considers itself to have long ago outgrown, for this natural healing principle is not new at all, but very old. Its beginnings coincide with the ancient beginnings of medicine itself.

4

An Ancient Principle Reasserts Itself

As far as historians can tell, the first person to propose a theory of healing based on the body's natural adaptive powers was the Greek physician Hippocrates, who lived around 400 B.C. He called those natural adaptive powers the *physis*, from which we get our word "physician." He described this *physis* as a "healing power," or a "self-adjusting power" within the body. "It is nature that finds the way," he wrote. "Though untaught and uninstructed, it does what is proper . . . to preserve a perfect equilibrium . . . to re-establish order and harmony."

A debate erupted. While Hippocrates carried the banner of the body's adaptive powers, the philosopher Democritus carried the banner of the unbelievers. He couldn't see how believing in this "healing power" differed from believing in the gods. Hippocrates allowed the healing power in his science because it was orderly and lawful. Democritus banished it from his science because it was invisible and unexplainable.

Democritus proposed instead a philosophy whose main point was that nature is nothing more than tiny particles that get combined and recombined. Everything in the universe, he argued, may be explained by referring to these particles — these "atoms" — and the forces that join them. What atoms and forces cannot explain, he declared, simply cannot be explained at all. He could envision within these particles no mystical "healing power."

These two opinions — one favoring the healing power, the other opposing it — were originally known as ***vitalism*** and *atomism*.

The debate between the two opinions has raged for nearly 2,500 years. In 300 A.D., the great physician Galen wrote, "There are two main schools in medicine and philosophy who have made any pronouncements about the nature of man." He referred to vitalism and atomism. Historian Harris Coulter wrote an 1,800-page, three-volume history of medicine that he called *Divided Legacy*, referring to the division in medical history between these two schools of thought, and tracing their debate through every era of history, including our own. Virtually every other medical history, as far as I've been able to discover, acknowledges this same division of thought.

Medicine Takes Sides in the Ancient Debate

When Benjamin Rush and his colonial colleagues decided to wrest healing from the body's adaptive powers, they were simply taking sides in this ancient debate. They didn't invent the issue, nor did they invent the arguments they used to justify their position. They became atomism's heirs by deliberate and conscious choice. As one historian put it, atomism became "an inspiring idea for the spiritual fathers of modern science," while "Hippocrates [with his vitalistic ideas] was dethroned as the scientific authority."

But vitalism didn't die. It was simply banished to a sort of scientific and philosophical underground. Homeopathy is a vitalist principle. So is the idea that foods can heal. Many herbal philosophies — Chinese herbalism in particular — come from vitalism. Chiropractic is vitalist, as is the new discipline of psychoneuroimmunology, which speaks of the mind's power to affect our health. Color therapy, music therapy, and humor therapy come from the vitalist tradition. Though these therapies differ widely, they share in common both their vitalist philosophy (all claim to be ways of enhancing the body's natural adaptability) and the fact that conventional medicine typically condemns them as unscientific, unproven, and "quackery."

Unscientific or not, the natural healing principle casts a profoundly different light on things. Even germs shift meaning. While medicine condemns germs as an enemy to be destroyed, the natural healing principle considers them simply living creatures we share this planet with, sometimes peacefully, sometimes not. When our adaptive powers are strong, we live with germs in peace, though we may become sick from time to time as a means of adapting to their presence. But when our adaptive powers become weak, those same germs remind us we've allowed ourselves to become less than we ought to be. They scourge us now, and motivate us to become strong again, which we may do by understanding and living wholesome principles. And while we may seek to destroy germs in a crisis, to eradicate them altogether would be pure foolishness. For while germs infect us when we're weak, they add to our strength when we're strong. They provoke our immune system, arouse it, cause it to grow, to become ever more powerful. Without germs, we'd have no immune powers at all, and we'd be absolutely susceptible should something unexpected happen along.

As for chemical imbalances, they simply become signs of the disorder and weakness we've brought upon ourselves by failing to live a healthy life. They can generally be reversed by the very principles that would have prevented them in the first place.

Differing Views on the Meaning of Disease

Perhaps nothing so differentiates the two philosophies as the way they view disease. Medical science seeks to fight disease, and to neutralize whatever it perceives to be disease's cause. The natural healing principle accepts disease as natural, inevitable, and even helpful, and focuses on understanding principles for strengthening our body's natural adaptive powers. In that sense, natural healing therapies *have nothing to do with curing disease*. They seek only to strengthen, not to oppose.

In fact, from the natural healing perspective, illnesses don't even exist — at least not in any practical sense — and certainly not as *disease entities* that we can give names to, which is the medical way of viewing things. In medicine, you can hardly start to work on an illness until you give it a name. In the case of AIDS, for example, nobody tried to find out what causes it, or how to treat it, until medical scientists decided they'd found a new disease. Even to talk about it, they had to name it, so they called it "Acquired Immune Deficiency Syndrome," and the disease list grew by one. Doctors discover new diseases more or less as botanists discover new plants.

The parallel between medicine and botany is more than coincidental. Classifying has always been the *conceptual* foundation of science. If you don't classify things, you don't know what they are. The Swedish botanist Carolus Linnaeus invented scientific classification, and published his first "taxonomy" of living things — a breakdown into kingdoms, phylums, classes, orders, etc. — in 1735. Less than forty years later, the Frenchman Francois Boissier de Sauvages published the first taxonomy of diseases, broken down in almost exactly the same way. He began with ten classes, divided them into forty orders, and finally ended up at the bottom with more than 2,400 "species" of diseases, each as real, in a scientific sense, as tulips or black-eyed Susans.

Today virtually everything about medicine hinges on the modern version of this taxonomy of diseases. The National Library of Medicine publishes a 470-page "tree structure" of medical subjects. Section C, which is 87 pages long, covers *Diseases*. Its entries look like this:

- Virus diseases
  - Arbovirus Infections
    - Encephalitis, Epidemic
      - Encephalitis, California
      - Encephalitis, Japanese B
      - Encephalitis, St. Louis
      - Encephalitis, Tick-borne
        - Louping Ill
      - etc.

"Virus diseases" is a main category; "Arbovirus Infections" is a subcategory; "Encephalitis, Epidemic" is a sub-sub-category; and so on. There's a branch of medicine called *nosology* that does nothing but name and classify diseases. The point is that diseases, for scientific purposes, are "entities," which the dictionary defines as "existing independently and apart from other things." If you and I both get "Japanese B Encephalitis," we get the same thing, and it exists entirely apart from us. That's why I can "give" it to you, or you can "get" it from me, as though we're exchanging Christmas gifts.

This is part of what makes medicine seem so impersonal. Although doctors may care for us at one level, at another level they must act as if we don't exist. What may be treated in the test tube, or in a rat, may also (almost coincidentally) be treated in a human body. Conceptually, the three circumstances are the same. The disease and the cure remain constant *across circumstances*, of which we are but one of an infinite number of possibilities. X drug kills Y disease, no matter who — or what — has it. Though doctors may personally wish it otherwise, they don't treat *us*, they treat the disease; nor do they concern themselves with the *general* state of our adaptive powers. Their training prohibits it.

And *that* is probably the key difference between natural healing and medicine. Natural healing focuses on the *general* state of our individual adaptive powers; medicine focuses on *specific* remedies for *specific* diseases that exist apart from individuals. The California Medical Association, in its booklet *The Professional's Guide to Health & Nutrition Fraud*, warns, "Be wary of claims that a product may be used for multiple health problems. Generally speaking, such products exist only in the portfolios of con artists." You can understand why they say that if you understand that, from the medical perspective, each disease on those 87 pages of the National Library of Medicine's tree structure has a separate cause and a separate cure, both external to the body.

From the natural healing perspective, however, all of those "diseases" (except those that are clearly genetic) boil down to the same thing — our adaptive powers are weak — and strengthening one or another aspect of those adaptive powers will handle any of the diseases. For that reason, we don't need to name diseases. Our adaptive powers don't stop working if we forget to tell them what they're fighting. And if we end up doing exactly the same healthful thing for a wide range of diseases (which in natural healing happens more often than not), the differences between those diseases literally don't exist in any practical sense. And in no case is what we do designed to *cure* anything. We do what makes us healthy, and the "cure" follows as a matter of course.

Drawing the Body into Balance

Virtually all natural healing therapies have as their goal to establish some sort of *balance*. For example, our immune system consists of two opposing forces: an attacking force, and a suppressing force. The attacking force includes the killer T cells, the B cells with their antibodies, and the cell-eating phagocytes. The suppressing force includes mainly the suppressor T cells. When we're invaded, the attacking cells rush to our defense with a sort of vicious-cycle explosiveness that could easily get out of hand. The suppressor cells somehow monitor that explosiveness and shut it off when the attack, like Goldilocks' porridge, is *just* right.

But suppose the attack isn't *just* right. It can get off balance in either of two ways: by being shut off (1) too late, or (2) too soon. In the first case, the attack is too strong. In the second case, the suppression is too strong. Since our immune system has to handle both foreign cells and our body's own cells, this leads to four possible out of balance conditions that coincide with four major categories of diseases, as Table 1 (next page) shows.

As you can see, too much *attack* against foreign cells leads to *allergies* like hay fever; too much attack against our own cells leads to *auto-immune conditions* like arthritis and diabetes. Too much *suppression* against foreign cells leads to *infections* like measles and the flu; too much suppression against our own cells leads to *tumors*.

From the medical point of view, each of these four categories, and each of the diseases within them, poses a separate problem, with a separate cause and a separate cure. The cures share in common, however, that they are *interventions*. With drugs, we either suppress the immune system to reduce its excess attack, attack our enemies to

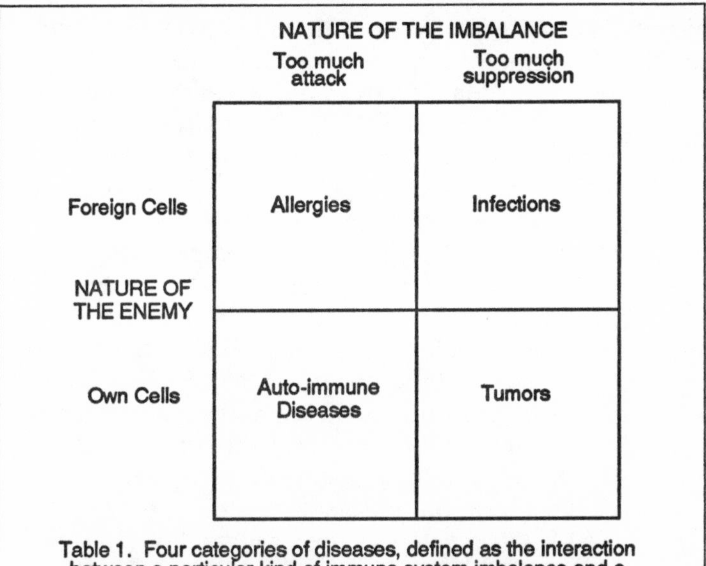

NATURE OF THE ENEMY	NATURE OF THE IMBALANCE: Too much attack	NATURE OF THE IMBALANCE: Too much suppression
Foreign Cells	Allergies	Infections
Own Cells	Auto-immune Diseases	Tumors

Table 1. Four categories of diseases, defined as the interaction between a particular kind of immune system imbalance and a particular kind of cell that the body is called upon to handle.

make up for its excess suppression, or we directly manipulate the chemical imbalances that we determine to be at fault. In other words, we do with drugs what the body fails to do for itself. What makes the whole thing complex is that, having decided to intervene, we must do it *at the body's level*, with roughly the same molecular precision that the immune system uses.

From the natural healing point of view, in contrast, the four cells and the diseases within them all represent the *same* problem: our body has gotten out of balance. And natural healing therapies share in common that they do *not* intervene, but rather seek to create conditions that allow the body to spontaneously move into balance again.

We Reflect the Quality of our Context

When we speak of "conditions," we refer to what we might call our "context," or our surroundings. Context becomes important because we, like all living things, are "open systems," meaning that we receive things from our context and *transform* them. In scientific terms, the things we receive from our context (food, water, air, etc.) are "fluxes." We can't live without them. As Nobel prize-winner Ilya Prigogine put it, open systems, whether cities or cells, "cannot be separated from the fluxes that they incessantly transform," or they will die. These fluxes from our context are so important, in fact, that *our* nature depends on *their* nature. As their quality changes, so does the quality of our life. Fluxes flow in; life flows out.

My office window overlooks a cherry tree. The cherry tree receives elements from its context — air, water, sunlight, chemicals from the soil, and so on — and transforms them into cherries. I, in turn, transform the cherries into my version of life, and the quality of my life shifts a bit to reflect the passing-through of those cherries. I am affected, not only by their nutrients, but by their beauty, and their taste, even by the grateful thoughts they inspire.

I can make a loop out of this sort of thing by spending a bit of the life I've created to affect the quality of my cherries. But to do so, I don't worry about the tree's biochemistry or its genes. Genes obviously make a difference — I'll get no better cherries than the tree's genes allow — but the tree's genes are more or less given, as they are with us. My challenge is to get from those genes the best that's in them. For that, I must create for my tree a healthful context. I nourish it, water it, even sing to it or give it love pats if I believe such things help. If pests attack, I may be inclined to try to kill them, but I know also that trees naturally *resist* pests. So while I do what I can to keep the pests away, most of all, I support my tree. I nurture it *contextually* to call forth the best possible expression of its genetic potential, of which pest-resistance is an inseparable part.

That, more or less, is the idea behind the natural healing principle. Our cells have a context, which is our *inner* context; we also have an *outer* context. Our body manages our inner context; we manage our outer context. The two are connected. Our outer context *becomes* our inner context. That's what it means to say we're *open* systems. To a degree, the body can overcome a poor outer context. It has processes for purifying the fluids that bathe the cells, balancing their constituents, managing their temperature, keeping them flowing, and so on. But it can only do so much. When we create a poor outer context for ourself, we at least make the body work harder, and at worst, we break it down. Conversely, as we heal our context, we very likely heal ourselves.

An All-encompassing Principle

What this means is that there are as many ways to apply the natural healing principle as there are aspects to our context. Food obviously enters here, as do water and air. As the quality of these life-sustaining elements increases, so does the quality of what they become, which is everything that we are. As pollutants degrade the quality of our context, they degrade *our* quality as well.

From this perspective, even the news we hear becomes an aspect of context. In an intriguing experiment, researchers dropped billfolds with $20 bills in them on the streets of New York City to see how many would get returned. The answer, they found, was nearly 50%. Except on one day. On that day, not a single billfold was returned. When the investigators sought to understand why, they discovered that Bobby Kennedy had been killed the night before. The shocking news apparently embittered the normally altruistic spirit of those who, on more joyful days, would have returned the money.

And *that*, in turn, probably affected the quality of their health. Nerves connect our brain to every part of our immune system. Any sort of mental stress instantly transforms itself into hormone shifts that have been linked to ill health. Research even shows that we can affect our health simply by choosing to see things from an optimistic point of view.

A Non-material Context?

As you can see, the body's context seems to include non-material things, like our thoughts. But how can non-material thoughts affect material processes? It seems impossible, but there's little doubt that they do.

Imagine, for example, a runner who's exhausted and stops to rest. We expect that resting will leave him stronger, and in some ways it does. But in other ways, resting leaves him *less* organized for running.

Here's why. To contract, the runner's muscle fibers have to have a high concentration of potassium on the inside, and a low concentration on the outside. While the runner runs, that concentration difference exists. But the instant he stops to rest, half the potassium leaks from inside the fiber to the outside, which destroys the concentration difference, and the muscle can't contract. The leaking that destroys the difference is driven by those disorganizing processes of entropy that we talked about.

Now, when the runner starts to run again, the potassium that leaked outside moves back into the fiber and recreates the concentration difference, which lets the muscle contract. The contractions after the rest are actually weaker than the contractions before the rest until that concentration difference builds up, and the muscle operates again at full capacity.

Now, what moves the potassium? What force shifts the outside potassium to the inside so the muscle can contract? As far as I can see, it began with a thought — the intention to run. The leaking that diffuses the potassium creates disorder and weakness. The thinking that restores the concentration creates order and strength. We have here what seems to be an instance of non-material intentions ordering material processes in the body. Is this how the placebo effect works?

System or Context?

We have two philosophies of health because, in a system that draws life from its context, order is the child of two parents: (1) the system itself, and (2) the context that sustains it. When we get sick, medicine blames the system and seeks to repair or replace it. Natural healing blames the context and seeks to make it more healthful.

In some cases —genetic disorders, for instance — the system is clearly at fault. In other instances, however, it's harder to say. Take cancer, for example. Is cancer a system breakdown? Or is it a context breakdown? Medicine calls it a system breakdown — the genes aren't working right. But the issue is by no means clear.

5

Two Briefs in the Case Against Cancer

According to conventional medical theory, cancer begins with a single cell whose genes have become damaged or deranged through some genetic accident. The damaged genes cause the cell to multiply out of control. The cell's descendants inherit the cancerous genes, and their growth overtakes and destroys the body's normal functions. Substances that damage genes are *carcinogens*. Theoreticians believe carcinogens may activate certain cancer-producing genes — called *oncogenes* — that remain dormant in normal cells. This explanation is only an assumption, however. Certain biological facts now argue against it.

For example, cancer theorists first assumed that normal cells turn into cancer cells in a single step. But cancer has turned out to be a *process* — a *series* of related changes. A single genetic accident seems reasonable; a series seems much less likely. Some theorists assume cancer cells are exceptionally unstable, or accident prone. Yet studies show they suffer genetic accidents or mutations no more often than normal cells.

The changes that lead to cancer appear to mimic a process called *gene amplification*. Cells amplify genes by making more of them. The extra genes cause the cell to produce extra amounts of certain chemicals, which cause the cell to multiply. According to cancer theorist Robert T. Schimke, gene amplification and the gene changes leading to cancer are "analogous processes."

Yet while cancer is abnormal, gene amplification is not. As Schimke puts it, "gene amplification is one of the most common phenomena in biology, and occurs in virtually all types of organisms." Another expert called gene amplification "pervasive," explaining that it occurs "with high frequency," and that it involves "a very large amount of DNA, probably including many genes."

An Adaptive Process

Not only is gene amplification common, it appears to be how living organisms adapt. For example:

- When cells receive high doses of toxic metals, they amplify genes that build up their resistance.
- Cells amplify resisting genes when they're exposed to repeated small doses of toxins, but not when they're exposed to a single large dose. If gene amplification were a genetic accident, the reverse would more likely be true.
- Genes amplify at a precise moment during cell division, and the process begins and ends at the same time at many locations throughout the gene.
- When a cell builds resistance, it amplifies genes for the human growth hormone and at least five other proteins that help regulate cell division.
- A number of important body chemicals, including insulin and interferon, encourage gene amplification.
- Cells that amplify genes when exposed to a single toxin may develop resistance to a number of unrelated toxins at the same time.
- When cells first experience toxins, they undergo a temporary gene amplification that goes away if the

toxin is removed. But if exposure continues, they undergo a second, more stable form of gene amplification that persists even after the toxin is removed.

- Gene amplification is the process by which bacteria resist antibiotics.

This evidence clearly suggests that gene amplification is a mechanism for adapting. If so, perhaps that analogous process we call cancer is itself an adaptation. This, of course, is what the natural healing principle suggests.

Organizing Fields

When we view cancer as an adaptation, we shift our attention from the cell to its context. Could an abnormal context cause a normal cell to lose control? Surprisingly, the answer is *Yes*.

Genes give a cell power to adapt, but they don't guide it. The information that guides a cell comes from its context. This has been true from the moment we were conceived.

We began as a single cell that divided, then redivided, again and again. In the process, we became trillions of cells. All of our cells have the same genes as the original, yet they do many different things. One cell senses light, another contracts when chemicals stimulate it, and so on. The differences obviously can't depend on the genes, since the genes in every cell are the same. Different cells do different things depending on which genes get *expressed*. Which genes get expressed depends on a cell's context.

For example, up to a certain point in an embryo's development, a skin cell transplanted to the eye becomes an eye cell, and vice versa. This has led scientists to talk about "organizing fields," or contexts that organize a cell's functions. Some scientists call these "individuation fields," since they lead cells to become individual, or unique.

When the organizing field is strong, the cell develops strongly and precisely. When the organizing field is weak, the cell develops weakly and without direction. The point is that the information that guides a cell's development, and later, its adaptation, comes from the outside — from the context, or organizing field, that surrounds it. Based on that information, the cell *integrates* with its context.

Organizing fields are strongest, it seems, where we most need to adapt. For example, certain lizards easily lose and regrow their tails, which is handy since the tail is where their large enemies are most likely to catch them. To regrow, those tail cells need a strong organizing field, and there's an exact point moving down a lizard from its head to its tail where the organizing field begins. If you plant a tumor cell on the tail side of that point, the organizing field transforms it into a normal tail cell. But if you transplant it on the head side of the point, it remains a tumor cell and multiplies without direction.

For a long time, people assumed that adult mammals (which don't regenerate limbs like lizards) didn't have organizing fields, that organizing fields happened only in mammal *embryos*, that they guided *development* before birth, but not *adaptation* after it. There's evidence now, however, that organizing fields operate in adults as well. In one experiment, for instance, scientists transplanted cells from a rat's kidney to its prostate gland, and the cells developed what the scientists called "prostatic activity." This is convincing evidence, they said, that even adult cells rely on information from their surroundings to keep themselves organized.

Losing the Beat

Cells get both chemical and electrical information from their surroundings, since the body communicates with both. Cells create electrical fields, for example. Two cells that sit within each other's fields create an electrical network. Changes in one cell's electrical field affect what goes on in the other cell, and vice versa. Since nerves also create electrical fields, a cell may also be influenced from farther away, by the brain or other parts of the nervous system. Electrical patterns may be precise and clear, or they may be distorted and disturbed, as anyone who listens to the radio can testify. As a cell's electrical context disorganizes, so do its genetic processes.

Cells also pass soluble chemicals back and forth from one to another through gaps or channels in their cell membranes. When those channels and their messages are blocked, embryo cells develop defects, which suggest that losing those messages lets their genetic processes get off track. The body's hormones (insulin, estrogen, cortisone, etc.) also affect cells, so chemicals, like electricity, also influence from afar.

In all of this, timing seems particularly important. The chemical levels inside a cell go up and down in cycles, as do both the electrical and chemical fields outside of the cell. The up and down rhythms "time" the cell, like a clock. Between chemistry and electricity, there may be hundreds, or even thousands, of rhythmic cycles, both inside and outside of the cell, all synchronized, all part of an intricate timing mechanism. If they get out of sync, the cell loses order and efficiency, like a car with bad timing, a band that loses the beat, or a basketball team that can't quite get in the flow of the game.

Cells Lose Control in a Weak Context

As you can see, cells need two things to work right: (1) good genes, and (2) a strong organizing context. Even the best genes lose control in a weak context.

For example, when scientists take healthy cells from the body and culture them in a dish, the cells stop doing what they did in the body, and begin to multiply out of control, just like cancer cells. Cells have "markers" that tell where they came from. Some of those markers start to disappear instantly, some last two days, some five days, some eight. After ten days or so, the cells no longer bear signs of what their function in the body might have been.

The changes that take place in these cultured cells are the very ones that turn normal cells into cancer cells. Cancer theorists blame them on mutations or genetic accidents. Yet they happen here with only a change in context. They are, in fact, changes in the genes, but they happen far too rapidly to be mutations. Mutations are relatively rare. These gene-changes appear to be *adjustments* to the new context, and they happen at least 100 times more rapidly than mutations.

Further evidence that these changes are no accident comes from the study of *karyotypes*. A cell's karyotype is the pattern or arrangement of its genes. Scientists who study karyotypes in cancer cells have concluded that "the karyotype profile of a tumor represents *an adaptation* of the cells to the particular environment in which they are multiplying," and "the changes observed [in tumor cells]...are not due to the selection of rare spontaneous mutations in the population *but appear to be adaptive*." (Italics added.)

All of this directly contradicts medicine's assumption that cancer cells have damaged or mutated genes. The same changes occur both in cancer cells within the body, and in normal cells that are separated from the body and raised in a dish. What can these two kinds of cells have in common but a weak or disorganized context?

Delay Can Make Disorder Permanent

In fact, when scientists take these cultured cells from their dishes and return them to their normal, healthy context within the body, they become normal, healthy cells. They regain their markers, they begin to make their proper chemicals, and they resume their relationship to the cells around them. Cancer cells taken from a cancerous animal and placed within the body of a healthy animal also return to normal.

But only up to a point. After so long in the disorganized context, the cell's adaptations to it become stable. In a study of cartilage cells, researchers found that the cells "quickly lose their capacities for making their specific products when they are dispersed, but regain them when they are packed together again. If they are kept in the dispersed state for more than ten days, however, reassociation fails to restore their function."

Another study concluded, "Cells that are clearly neoplastic [cancerous], even to the point of metastasizing [spreading], will lose their malignant character when those initial conditions are removed [when they're placed in a normal animal, in other words]; if the conditions persist long enough, however, the cells gain the capacity to form tumors in a normal host."

Both quotes are a bit obscure, but the point they make is the same: if cells stay too long without the guidance of a strong organizing context, they end up unable to be guided at all. The adaptation becomes much more difficult to reverse.

Resisting Chemotherapy

With this background, let's consider what chemotherapy does. Chemotherapy is toxic. Its purpose is to ***kill*** cells. Doctors operate with the hope, therefore, that they can find a chemotherapy that will kill cancer cells and leave normal cells alone. But if cancer cells are *normal* cells whose *context* is abnormal, can you see how hopeless that aspiration is, particularly since chemotherapy simply adds one more abnormality to the context?

In fact, cells react to chemotherapy exactly as they react to any other toxin: by resisting it. And they resist chemotherapy through the very adaptive process that Robert T. Schimke described as analogous to cancer: *gene amplification*. In the very moment that chemotherapy seeks to destroy cancer cells, those cells respond by amplifying their genes to become more strongly cancerous.

For example, researchers exposed human cells to chemotherapy and saw a 250- to 350-fold amplification of the genes that help the cell divide. Other researchers did the same thing and saw that the chemotherapy "dramatically" increased gene amplification. And when drugs are combined (as they frequently are), gene amplification "is far greater (100 times) than predicted from the frequencies as determined separately for each drug."

These cancer cells are *resisting*. As doctors seek to kill them, they seek to stay alive. And they become stronger for doing so.

This is adaptation, *and* it is cancer. The two processes, in this instance, appear to be the same. By provoking adaptation to their chemotherapy, doctors literally provoke cancer. According to medical literature, chemotherapy (1) "stimulates tumor viability," (2) "gives a growth advantage to the tumor," and (3) "is associated with shortened survival" for the patient. Schimke himself concludes by asking, "Might such treatments convert relatively benign tumors into . . . more lethal form?"

On a Plateau

Cancer theorists admit they're stumped. "We're currently on a plateau," says Paul V. Woolley III of Georgetown University in Washington D.C. "There's a widespread feeling among people in the cancer field that further treatment gains will be a result of a much more detailed understanding of neoplastic [cancer] cells and an understanding of the mechanism by which the cells can adapt to and resist neoplastic drugs."

Even Schimke, whose research has begun to uncover the mechanism of resistance, doesn't interpret resistance as reason to abandon chemotherapy. On the contrary, he recommends simply that doctors use it more forcefully. "The doses of drugs should be sufficient that an effective concentration is delivered to result in cell death," he says. After all, only survivors develop resistance.

Yet if doctors can become more powerful, so can cells. While cells meet small drug doses by amplifying their genes, they meet stronger doses with an altogether different mechanism: *reduced binding affinity*, meaning they keep the drug from binding to the enzymes it affects. Beyond that lies still another resistance mechanism: *altered transport*, meaning they affect how the drug moves into the cell. Beyond that may lie still other defenses we don't even know about. These are the very processes that healthy cells use to preserve themselves. Doctors hope to understand them in order to break them down.

By medical logic, our victory in the war on cancer depends on winning this biological arms race. Yet if the logic of natural healing is correct, the search for stronger weapons misses the point. Our enemy in cancer is not the cells, but the context we've created for them. By the logic of natural healing, chemotherapy simply pollutes an already unhealthful context, which can only make the problem worse.

Testing the Explanations

This gives us a way to test the two explanations. The medical explanation predicts chemotherapy will heal cancer victims by killing their cancer. The natural healing explanation predicts chemotherapy will harm cancer victims by making their cancer worse. On this point, medical literature seems to support the natural healing explanation.

But scientists tend not to be persuaded, at least not to the point of accepting natural healing remedies. This is because natural healing remedies involve managing our context, and context includes *everything.* This all-encompassing property of the natural healing principle produces a certain fuzziness of detail that classically trained scientists find intolerable.

For example, suppose we discover an ill person who's been living virtually alone in an unkempt, darkened room. We move him to a bright, clean, comfortably furnished room, where we support him with warm, friendly people, feed him with nourishing food, comfort him with pleasant music, and entertain him with humorous stories. Suppose we massage him to improve his circulation and soothe his stiffened muscles. Suppose we even induce him to exercise a bit, or to read, or paint, or sing. In human terms, these sorts of things are more or less akin to caring for the context of the cherry tree. If a cherry tree can reflect the quality of its context in its cherries, might not our patient reflect the quality of his context in his health? According to the natural healing principle, the answer is *Yes*.

But to what do we attribute the change? Was it the food? The music? The fresh air? The cleanliness? Did he become more hopeful? If we claim our effort at natural healing helped, the classically trained scientist is likely to ask, "But can you *prove* it?" And we are likely to find ourselves stumped, because there's really nothing we can say that will satisfy the classical definition of scientific proof. So we give as evidence the patient himself. "Look at him," we say. "Check his vital signs. He's better, can't you see?" Our principle won't allow us to manipulate, nor to credit, any single element to the exclusion of the others. Yet that is exactly what the classically trained scientist requires.

What the classically trained scientist requires, in fact, is *double-blind studies*, and on this point these debates tend to hinge. "The matter is really quite simple," the classical scientist says. "Show me a well-designed double-blind study and I'll believe." Yet telling advocates of natural healing they have to prove themselves with double-blind studies is like telling Baptists they have to get baptized Catholics. It *sounds* simple, but simplicity is hardly the point.

6

Medicine and the Context of Helplessness

The essential element of the double-blind study is the *placebo*. A placebo is a neutral substance that looks, tastes, feels, and smells like the drug being tested. The only difference is, the drug affects the body; the placebo doesn't.

To conduct a double-blind study, researchers create two groups of people and match them in every possible way. The two groups, in other words, are virtually identical. To one group they give the drug; to the other they give the placebo. The study becomes "double-blind" because the researchers tell neither the doctor nor the patient whether the patient is receiving the placebo or the drug.

From the natural-healing perspective, the problem with double-blind studies is the context they create. That context denies the patient information, and subjects him to experimental control. By the logic of double-blindness, the patient is passive and powerless. The drug acts *upon* the patient; the patient acts not at all.

Natural healing holds that the patient's acting is *part* of the therapy. No natural healing principle justifies deceiving patients, or acting *upon* them, or controlling them from the outside. Controlling and healing are opposites, in fact, since we are fully healed only when we have become fully free.

The idea that we can't heal by controlling has certain scientific support. *Acting* and *being acted upon* literally create two distinct physiologies, with only the physiology of acting leading to health.

The Physiology of Helplessness

In scientific literature, the state of being acted upon is called "helplessness." We're helpless when we sense we can't control what happens to us, that our circumstances are controlling us. Scientists know how to create helplessness in animals, and they observe it in humans. In either case, they detect clear physiological disturbances that seem to accompany this state of helplessness.

To create helplessness in an animal, scientists subject it to some kind of *inescapable* stress. After so long, the animal literally undergoes a physiological shift, almost like throwing a switch. Several kinds of body chemicals become disturbed, and the immune system weakens. Studies show the presence of this helpless physiology in many diseases, including cancer, diabetes, high blood pressure, arthritis, PMS, Alzheimer's disease, depression, anorexia, bulimia, autism, schizophrenia, and epilepsy.

Scientists have done a number of studies to determine what causes the shift. They describe it as "the induction of anxiety or fear," and they point to one key element that seems to account for it more than any other. That element is *uncontrollability*, in which "the subject is not permitted to alter or exert control over the aversive event to which it is exposed." Uncontrollability is an element of *context*, and we respond to it with an unhealthful physiology of helplessness.

Provoking the Physiology of Helplessness

How might we respond, therefore, to the context of medicine in which the doctor controls and we submit? We know that the simple act of getting our blood pressure read can cause it to rise. How are we affected by long waits in waiting rooms filled with sick people? Or by a hospital routine that sets for us the smallest details of our existence? Is it possible that conventional medicine's most fundamental principle — the doctor's *mastery* of nature — actually creates a controlling context that is in itself unhealthful?

Norman Cousins wrote a book called *The Healing Heart*. He'd written an earlier book called *Anatomy of an Illness* that told how he got over a usually fatal connective tissue disease by lifting his spirits with humor, and by taking lots of vitamin C. In *The Healing Heart*, Cousins describes how he used the same sorts of principles to recover from a near-fatal heart attack.

At one point in the story, he takes a treadmill test. The doctor looks at the results and tells him he's got to have immediate heart bypass surgery. Cousins disagrees. He's been walking distances the test results suggest are impossible, which doesn't make sense to him. Either he's well enough to walk, or he's not.

Cousins refuses the surgery, ponders the situation, then tells his doctor he wants to take the test again. This time, however, *he* — Norman Cousins — will control the treadmill, and he requests that the test be administered in pleasant, non-clinical surroundings. Under those conditions, he retakes the test, and now the results show his heart is recovering. He doesn't need the operation.

In the first test, the treadmill controlled Cousins within a cold, clinical context. In the second test, Cousins controlled the treadmill within a pleasant, non-clinical context. Yet that difference so profoundly altered his physiology that under one circumstance he needed the surgery; under the other he didn't. The doctor's motives were entirely honorable, yet he proposed to operate on Cousins for a "heart condition" that he himself created with the design of his test.

Can Double-blind Studies Prevent Therapies From Working?

Now let's consider whether the same sort of external control might not also affect the outcome of experiments.

Let's compare two studies of vitamin C and cancer, one double-blind, the other not. Again, "double-blind" means half the patients take vitamin C; half take a placebo. Only the experimenter knows who's getting what.

In the *non*-double-blind study, Ewan Cameron and Linus Pauling, history's only winner of two unshared Nobel Prizes, gave 10 grams of vitamin C every day to 100 terminal cancer patients. They matched these patients in sex, age, and type of tumor with 1000 other patients who received nothing. The patients who received vitamin C survived 210 days, on the average, compared with 50 days for the patients who received nothing. Eighteen of the treated patients remained alive at the end of the study period; sixteen recovered completely. None of the untreated patients survived. Cameron and Pauling concluded that "this simple and safe form of medication [vitamin C] is of definite value in the treatment of patients with advanced cancer."

Other researchers disagreed with that conclusion and did a double-blind test to prove their point. They gave 60 patients 10 grams daily of vitamin C. They gave a matched group of 63 patients a placebo. None of the patients knew what they were getting, nor did their doctors. Both groups survived an average of 51 days; one patient in the placebo group remained alive at the end of the study period. A second double-blind study showed similar results. From this, experts conclude that "vitamin C has no role in the treatment of cancer."

So who's right? Let's assume both studies were done exactly as reported. We have honest research, therefore, on four treatment conditions for patients with terminal cancer. (1) Cameron and Pauling's vitamin C treatment, (2) no treatment, (3) double-blind vitamin C treatment, and (4) double-blind placebo treatment. Table 2 summarizes the results.

Why did the Cameron/Pauling vitamin C treatment produce results? Vitamin C alone didn't do it, because the double-blind vitamin C group got the same thing, and not only did everybody in that group die, they died four times faster than the Cameron/Pauling group. To figure out what produced the results, we've got to see how the two treatment groups differed.

	# of Subjects	Ave. time of Survival	# Alive at End of Study	# Who Recovered
Cameron/Pauling Vitamin C Treatment	100	210 days	18 (18%)	16 (16%)
No Treatment	1000	50 days	0 (0%)	0 (0%)
Double-Blind Vitamin C Treatment	60	51 days	0 (0%)	0 (0%)
Double-blind Placebo Treatment	63	51 days	1 (1.6%)	0 (0%)

Table 2. Comparison of results of four cancer treatment programs, taken from two studies — one double-blind, the other not — of vitamin C in cancer treatment.

There are at least two differences, both of which have to do with context: (1) The physicians in the Cameron and Pauling group believed in their therapy, and were trying to strengthen their patients' natural resistance. Doctors in the double-blind group didn't even know what their therapy was; they were blindly handing out undefined pills. (2) Cameron and Pauling involved the patients by telling them what was going on; researchers in the double-blind study deliberately kept the patients from knowing what was happening to them.

These differences in approach could account for the differences in the results. To see why, look at Figure 1, which I've adapted from the book, *The Stress of Life*, by Hans Selye. It shows three stages in adapting to stress.

The first stage is the "Alarm Reaction." Notice these two things about the Alarm Reaction: (1) the line at the top of the diagram has a hump, which shows that the body is producing lots of *corticoid* hormones (cortisone and cortisol are corticoid hormone); (2) all of the lines in the box (which represent different body systems) are darkened, which means the whole body is *aroused*, yet no system is adapting. During this stage, the immune system is basically shut off.

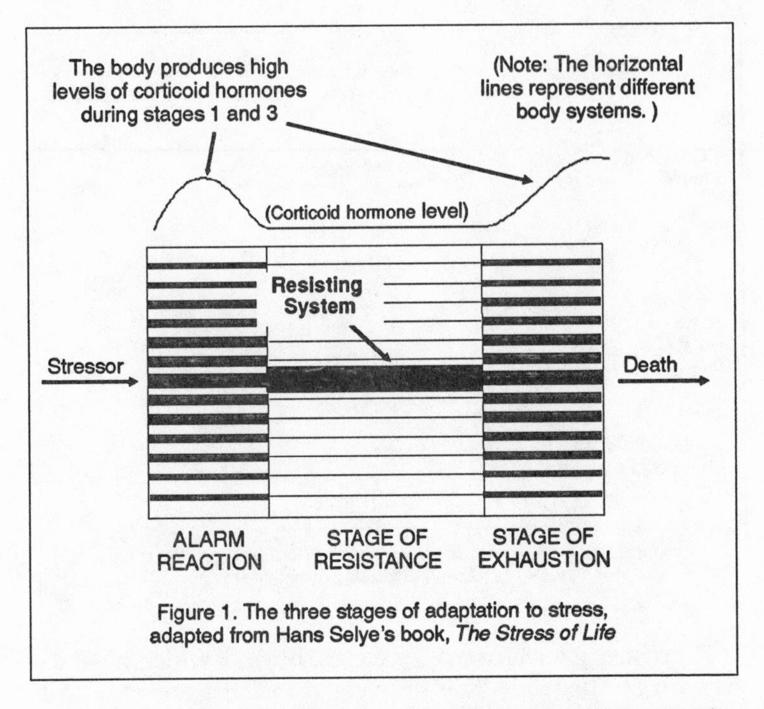

Figure 1. The three stages of adaptation to stress, adapted from Hans Selye's book, *The Stress of Life*

The second stage is "Resistance." In this stage: (1) the line at the top has flattened, which shows that the body no longer overproduces the corticoid hormones; and (2) only one line is darkened, which means the body is *adapting* by putting all of its resources into the single system that's best equipped to resist. In the case of cancer, that's the immune system.

The third stage is "Exhaustion." This appears to coincide with the switch to helplessness that accompanies the perception of uncontrollabilty. Physiologically, exhaustion is like the Alarm Reaction: the body produces high levels of corticoids; all systems get aroused, but none adapt. The immune system shuts off here as well.

Research on vitamin C shows it does two things that relate to this diagram. (1) It helps regulate the production of the corticoid hormones; (2) it helps regulate the immune response. If you look again at the diagram, you'll see that the corticoid hormones get triggered in stages 1 and 3. The immune system turns on only during stage 2.

Within these three stages we have two opposite and mutually exclusive reactions. Stages 1 and 3 represent a stress reaction that's most likely tied to the experience of uncontrollabilty and helplessness that we talked about in the last section. Alarm is the stress of uncertainty; exhaustion is the stress of defeat. Corticoids are *stress* hormones. They're prominent in the physiology of helplessness, and they actually *depress* the immune system, which helps explain the link between stress and illness.

Stage 2 represents adaptation, or resistance. Only in this stage does the body mobilize those immune system cells that fight cancer.

Vitamin C gets used in either reaction. But we can't predict what it will get used for, nor its effect, until we know which stage a person is in.

Logically, we would expect terminal cancer patients to be in the Stage of Exhaustion. If that's true, we should find them high in corticoids, low in resistance, which is indeed the case. One study showed a dramatic increase in corticoid production within the six months before death, which matches Selye's diagram exactly. Another study showed direct links between corticoids and cancer — patients were higher in corticoids than non-patients; their corticoid levels went up as their cancer got worse, down as their cancer got better.

If patients remain in the Stage of Exhaustion, giving them vitamin C won't necessarily affect their immune system. It will help modulate the corticoid hormones, which affects their stress response, and may *indirectly* affect their immune system. But to directly affect their immune system, we've got to get them out of the Stage of Exhaustion and into the Stage of Resistance.

According to Selye, which stage those cancer patients are in depends, in part at least, on their mental state — on how they're taking their cancer. There's a certain *emotional* resistance that accompanies physiological resistance. If we can somehow tip their emotional and physiological balance toward resistance, we'll also tip their vitamin C from stress hormones to the immune system, where it might actually do their cancer some good.

So which way does the emotional context of a double-blind study tip the balance? Double-blind studies deliberately keep patients in a state of uncertainty and helplessness. The very purpose of double-blindness is to eliminate emotional factors and isolate the pure and uncontaminated effect of the vitamin C. But vitamin C has no pure and uncontaminated effect. Its effect depends on the very emotional factors that the double-blind design seeks to eliminate. In the two studies we're considering, isn't it possible, perhaps even likely, that the double-blind design kept patients in a state of uncontrollability where they used their vitamin C, not to fight cancer, but to modulate the stress response? Could that be why the vitamin C seemed not to effect their cancer?

Cameron and Pauling refused to place their patients in the uncertainty of double-blindness. They openly sought to build their immune system. They involved their patients by telling them what they were getting. Isn't is possible, perhaps even likely, that some of those patients responded to that encouragement by moving from the Stage of Exhaustion into the Stage of Resistance where their vitamin C found use doing its job in the immune system? Could that be why nearly one-fifth of them survived?

We may question whether the context set by the design of a test could so drastically affect people's physiology. One study found that the anxiety of taking an academic test significantly weakened the immune system of medical students. Another study found that people experienced "changes in protein, carbohydrate, vitamin metabolism, heart rate, [and] adrenal function" when they did nothing more than *anticipate* a stressful situation. If these fairly normal activities can so profoundly alter physiology, it seems possible that the uncertainty of the double-blind design, particularly when coupled with the inherent impersonality of most medical settings, could likewise affect the physiology of cancer patients.

And in any of these settings, might not a context of openness and human caring *reduce* anxiety, and therefore affect adaptive responses for the better? Perhaps that's what happened in the Cameron/Pauling study, and what did *not* happen in the double-blind design. Physiological research suggests that vitamin C would be called into play in either case, but in only one of the two settings would it go toward fighting cancer.

This is all speculation, of course. But it fits certain biological facts, and it probably accounts for the results of these conflicting studies as well as any explanation. (Opponents of the Cameron/Pauling study say the positive results came from "selection bias," a point of view that's even *more* speculative, since they offer no evidence for it other than their disagreement.) If the explanation I've presented here is correct, it says that some double-blind patients died *because of the design of the test*. The design of the test *prevented* a therapy from working, rather than proving it didn't work.

No "Paradigm" May Demand that Other Paradigms Meet its Standards of Proof

In scientific terms, medicine and natural healing are competing *paradigms* (pronounced pair-a-dimes), or ways of explaining things. As Thomas Kuhn points out in his *Structure of Scientific Revolutions*, paradigms, by virtue of *how* they explain, require, or allow, certain things, while they prohibit, or disallow, others. Those "things" that paradigms may require or disallow include what they define as important, how they measure things, the kinds of tests they use, the ethical principles that guide them, and in particular, the nature of their therapies. To be "scientific," a paradigm must be consistent *within itself*, and it must prove useful. No paradigm may be judged wrong simply because it violates the requirements and prohibitions of its competitor.

By the nature of its explanations, medicine allows — even requires — a treadmill test in which the doctor controls the patient, and research studies in which both patients and doctors are kept blind. Natural healing prohibits such things because they create an unhealthful context.

Classically trained scientists typically demand that advocates of natural healing prove their therapies with double-blind studies. Yet no principle of science suggests that a single paradigm may somehow rule over all others, or that a single paradigm may require that all others meet *its* standards of proof. In fact, there are good reasons for questioning whether the double-blind standard of scientific proof works even for medicine itself.

7

The Perils of Double-blindness

Double-blind studies are supposed to test safety and effectiveness. Yet studies have shown adverse drug reactions in more than ten percent of children visiting a group pediatric practice. Did the double-blind studies of those drugs show those reactions? If not, how can we conclude that the studies are valid? If the studies *did* show the reactions, why were the drugs approved? Is ten percent adverse reactions in our children an acceptable medical risk?

Tardive dyskinesia is a drug side-effect — a movement disorder marked by involuntary twitching of the mouth, lips, tongue, arms, legs or trunk. According to *Science News*, "somewhere between 15 percent and 25 percent of psychiatric patients treated with neuroleptic drugs develop tardive dyskinesia," which "has been basically untreatable." Neuroleptic drugs are supposed to treat mental disorders. But every time psychiatrists use them, they run roughly a one-in-five risk that they're going to give the patient an untreatable movement disorder. Did these statistics show up in the double-blind studies?

Another problem, apart from whether or not double-blind studies work, is that doctors sometimes use drugs for things they haven't been tested for. As *Science News* points out, neuroleptic drug treatment "is also widely used with the retarded to control behavior problems, *although there is little research on its effectiveness in such cases*" (italics added). With retarded patients, the proportion that gets tardive dyskinesia rises to one-in-three.

We Can't Eliminate All Possible Explanations

The idea behind double-blind studies is to eliminate every possible explanation for your results except the one you're trying to test. For example, suppose you give a drug to one group, and a placebo to another. The people in the drug group all get better, so you conclude that the drug works. But the "drug group" was all women, and the "placebo group" was all men. Maybe the women got better just because they were women. You didn't design the study to eliminate gender as a possible explanation.

So you do the study again. This time you mix the genders, randomly assigning equal numbers of men and women to both groups. That way, if the drug group gets better, you will have eliminated the explanation that it was gender that did it.

That sort of thing, as I mentioned earlier, is called "matching your groups." You try to make the two groups as alike as possible. Any variable on which the groups *differ* may be a possible cause of whatever your results turn out to be. Any variable on which the groups are the same *cannot* be a cause.

So you very carefully match your two groups, making sure they're identical on things like age, sex, education, economic class, and so on, and making sure you do your experimental procedures exactly the same for both groups. Remember, anything the groups differ on can be a possible cause, so you have to get rid of all the differences except the one you're trying to test.

The problem is, that's impossible. There's simply no way to perfectly match the groups, so you can't perfectly eliminate all of the alternative explanations. Also, that much control creates such an artificial situation, one that tests such a narrow range of things, that you'd have to conduct virtually an infinite number of studies to cover all of the possibilities.

For example, suppose you do a perfect double-blind study. You match your groups, create a perfect placebo, administer the drug to Group A, the placebo to Group B, with identical procedures. You determine that the drug has a particular effect, with a particular toxicity. You publish your results, and the drug gets approved.

But there's a problem. Both the effect of drugs and their toxicity vary, depending on the time of day. This is because our body's chemical levels go up and down during the day. A drug can be several times more effective, or more toxic, at one time during the day than another.

So you re-do the study. This time you do 24 studies, administering both the drug and the placebo at a different hour in each study. Now you know how the safety and effectiveness of the drug vary with the time of day, and you feel confident you can teach doctors how to use it.

But there's yet another problem. Those up and down cycles of our body chemicals vary depending on our age. Newborns don't show an endorphin cycle, for example. Old people's cycles tend to be shallower. Teenagers have odd cycles because they're going through puberty, and so on. So now you run 168 studies (24 hours-of-administration by 7 stages-of-the-life-cycle), and at last you understand all of the drug's side-effects and benefits as they relate to time-of-administration and age-of-the-patient.

There's more. Studies show, for example, that the food we eat can alter the biological effects of a drug. So we really ought to test the drug against different diets. And so on.

Double-blind Studies Miss the Second Phase

Suppose we could design a perfect series of double-blind studies to check out all the possible confounding variables. We would still have a problem. Drugs tend to have a two-phased effect, as I mentioned earlier. (Remember the examples of the athletes who take steroids, and the idea of blocking endorphins in Sudden Infant Death babies?) Phase one is what the drug does to the body (lets the athlete build more muscles; lowers the baby's endorphin level); phase two is how the body adapts to the drug (the athlete produces less natural testosterone; the infant produces extra endorphin).

This sort of thing is the rule rather than the exception. It's the resistance principle that we talked about earlier. Some blood pressure drugs work by blocking the system that cause blood pressure to rise. This in turn generally triggers what one study called "vigorous compensatory activation" of the same system. The same principle explains how chemotherapy provokes cancer: the chemotherapy drug blocks the tumor's growth; the tumor compensates by accelerating its growth.

If we can generalize from the chemotherapy studies, these adaptive changes we call resistance take place at the level of our genes. Our body responds to the drug by either "amplifying" genes, or reducing genes, in order to produce more or less of whatever body chemicals it must adjust to counter the effect of the drug. Given enough time, these changes become permanent, or at least stable. These second-phase adaptive responses therefore represent the *true* physiological effect of the drug.

How can we be sure a double-blind study has tested the second phase of a drug's effect? When drugs are given throughout the course of the study, which is often the case, we can be virtually sure that the study has *not* tested the second-phase effects, because the drug tends to *mask* them. And if we give the drug, then withhold it, hoping to observe the second-phase effects, we can't be sure, even if we don't see any, that they won't show up later.

Perhaps this is why drugs so often get approved, then are recalled as their harmful long-term effects become apparent through experience. It would be interesting to list all of the drugs that have been recalled for being harmful, find out why they were recalled, and then see how often, with the aid of hindsight, we could now design a practical double-blind study that could be guaranteed to reveal the harmful effect. I would wager we would find it, more often than not, impossible.

An Unnatural Way to Learn

The problem with double-blind studies is that they're unnatural. We simply don't learn that way. The idea behind double-blind studies is to hold virtually everything constant, vary *only* the experimental variable, and see what varies with it. In real life, we do just the opposite. In real life, *everything* varies, and we notice what stays constant. We interact with a friend, whose acts and expressions vary infinitely. Yet we notice certain constant traits that we call his "personality." We observe a cup as it rotates through an unending series of turns and tumbles. Yet, though the impression that strikes our eye varies infinitely, the constant features that define the object's "cupness" remain forever apparent to us. This discerning of *constancies* isn't logical. We can't explain it. We can't teach it to our children. It's unscientific. But we all do it. And it's the opposite of the double-blind principle.

I once looked up the origin of the word "intelligence." It comes from a root that means "to gather." So we gather: we notice this, and we notice that, caring not at all to eliminate things or keep things that might confuse us from varying. We simply gather, which I take to mean that we *observe*. Then this brain of ours sorts through the variation, discovers the constant features, and these become the truths that, because of their constancy, we dare to rely on.

Double-blind experimental studies, with their checks and controls, properly belong to medicine, with *its* checks and controls. And they suffer, therefore, the same weakness: the "control" they claim is an illusion. I would wager that we haven't even been *designed* to control, since being able to control would take away our need to adapt. Adapting is so clearly part of our nature, and it seems so much more *peaceable* than controlling. If we haven't been designed to control, it shouldn't surprise us that we do it so poorly. We *have* been designed to *observe*, to *discern*, and to *adapt*, however, so it shouldn't surprise us that we do them so well.

8

Experience Is the Better Test

Since double-blind studies don't fit the natural-healing principle, what we know of natural-healing therapies generally comes from experience. This is called "empirical" knowledge, which the dictionary defines as "guided by practical experience and not theory, especially in medicine."

Medicine looks down on experience just as natural healing looks down on double-blind experiments. For example, one medical historian describes natural-healing therapies as "empiric in the derogatory sense." Another claims to see "a harmonious correlation between imagination, demonic activity, empirical observation, and naturalistic explanations."

Both quotes are rather obscure, so let me explain them by showing what they have in common. Keep in mind that "empiric" means "based on practical experience."

The author of the first quote — the one about natural healing being "empiric in the derogatory sense" — explains in the next sentence what he means. His complaint about experience is that what it teaches us is "based on correlations but devoid of an account of the relation between the phenomena correlated." What he wants, he says, is an "account of the relationship," by which he means an *explanation*, which experience alone doesn't provide.

I remember flipping a light switch once just as something went "bang!" in another part of the house. The two events — flipping the switch and the bang! — were so *correlated* that I had the eerie sense that my flipping the light switch had caused the bang. Suppose I tell that to you, and you, skeptic that you are, don't believe my flipping the switch had anything to do with the bang. You believe it was simple *coincidence* (which my dictionary defines as "an accidental sequence of events that appear to have a causal relationship"). You might ask me to convince you by giving "an account of the relationship." In other words, if I can tell you *how* flipping the switch caused the bang, then maybe you'll believe me. The problem with experience, this author is saying, is that it shows only "correlations," or "associations" between events, not what causes what. Associations let us *assume* two events are connected (I *assumed* that flipping the switch caused the bang), but nothing more. The scientific antidote for assuming is *explaining*. If we can explain a connection, chances are we'll believe it.

The author of the second quote complains about exactly the same thing. He sees "a harmonious correlation between imagination, demonic activity, empirical observation, and naturalistic explanations." What he means is that, when people rely on nothing more than their experience, they're likely to *explain* what they see by imagining all sorts of strange and unscientific things.

That happens, of course, so in a certain sense, what these authors say is correct. But in another sense, they miss the point. When we're trying to heal, how we *explain* things doesn't matter.

Explaining Isn't What Makes Things Work

For example, an article that condemned chiropractic carried the subtitle, "Spinal manipulation can be useful, but chiropractic's theoretical basis is a strange and never-demonstrated notion of subluxations." Imagine a doctor saying to a patient, "I wouldn't go to that chiropractor if I were you. I agree that his spinal manipulations are useful, but his theories are nonsense." What does the patient care, as long as the therapy works?

For another example, the author of an article in the *Journal of the American Medical Association*, while admitting that acupuncture works, praised recent studies "by reputable investigators [that] give an explanation for a mechanism of acupuncture that is in accord with modern scientific thinking as opposed to the *fanciful theories* of traditional Chinese medicine" (italics added). Again, the therapy already worked, but it didn't become "scientific" until the theories behind it made sense.

For a third example, in 1983, the *Los Angeles Times* reported a study done at the University of Texas that tested the effect of Chinese herbs against cancer. The article quoted the project director as saying, "We have something that works, or at least seems to. Our problem, however, is that *we do not know why or how it works*, and until we do, we cannot develop this as a modern medicine" (italics added).

Classical science assigns little value to knowing simply that something works. It assigns a much higher value to knowing *how* something works. As a result, it's scientifically possible, perhaps even required, to call a therapy "unscientific" or "unproven" simply because scientists don't know *how* it works, even if there's evidence that it *does* work, and even though knowing how something works doesn't change it's *therapeutic* value.

An Example of Demanding Too Much Proof

A few years ago, the R.J. Reynolds Tobacco Company ran several magazine ads claiming there's no conclusive scientific evidence that cigarettes cause disease. When the first ad came out, promising as it did an "open debate about smoking," *Science 84* magazine ran a skeptical editorial that it called "Behind a Smoke Screen." We don't know what the ads will say, the editorial said, "but it's a good bet they will use the same arguments the [tobacco] industry has proffered for 20 years." Those arguments go roughly like this:

> The studies that show smokers have higher risk than nonsmokers of contracting diseases are purely statistical. And statistics can't prove cause and effect. "The same thing that is wrong with the first study is wrong with the thirty thousandth," says a representative of the Tobacco Institute. "It just shows an association, not causation." Even in the case of lung cancer, says Charles Sommers, scientific director of the industry-funded Council for Tobacco Research, no laboratory animal, when forced to smoke, consistently develops the diseases associated with smoking in humans. Until a mechanism is found to explain how smoking leads to these illnesses, tobacco cannot be blamed.

You'll notice that the argument here is the same classical-science argument presented in the two quotes that began the chapter: the evidence "shows an association, not causation," and until we can "explain" the relationship, we haven't proven anything. The scientific argument that keeps natural healing therapies out of the marketplace keeps cigarettes *in* the marketplace. Cigarettes are legal because nobody can prove they harm us; herbs are illegal because nobody can prove they help us, at least not by the standards of classical science.

The problem here is not with cigarettes and herbs, but with the standard of proof set up by the tobacco industry and by those who oppose natural healing. It's so strict that it can't be met. You can't do a double-blind study of smoking because there's no placebo for a cigarette. And while you can do a double-blind study of an herb, the natural healing principle, which honors the patient's active self-reliance, forbids it. Herbs suffer the added drawback of being *complex*. You can't quite be sure what you've got when you use an herb. Herb species vary from region to region, and even within a single field, plants of a single species may vary in quality. Herbs come with too many uncertainties to ever be confirmed, to the satisfaction of those who oppose them, by the strict scientific standards that govern double-blind studies, which, in any case, can't be carefully enough controlled to conclusively prove anything.

Experience Gains Power as it Accumulates

What we're left with for testing natural products, then, is experience of the sort that allows us to conclude cigarettes cause cancer. The thing that gives experience its power is that it *accumulates*. I flip the light switch and something bangs. I get an eerie feeling — *perhaps flipping the switch caused the bang*. I flip the switch again. *Bang*! And again. *Bang*! The more I experience the association, the more I come to rely on it. Before long, the eerie feeling would come only if I *didn't* hear the bang, in which case I would suspect, even without explanations, that some *connection* had broken down.

As for double-blind studies, no amount of careful controlling can compensate for the fact that they *don't* accumulate. Classical science perpetrates a myth called "replication," in which someone allegedly repeats a study just to be sure of the results. Replication is a myth because "the modern biomedical research system is structured to prevent replication — not ensure it. It appears to be impossible to obtain funding for studies that are largely duplicative." So reports an author in *The New England Journal of Medicine*.

Scientific medicine itself proves without question that experience outweighs experiment. Suppose we ask of a newly approved drug, "What are its side effects?" Though double-blind studies just "proved" it safe and effective, the most truthful answer is probably, "We won't know until we actually use it." Doctors prescribe it, and a pattern of severe side effects shows up. Now double-blind experiments say one thing, experience says another. Wouldn't scientists lose their credibility if they insisted, in this circumstance, that double-blind experiments are the better test of truth?

When we observe associations that persist across time and circumstances, we're obliged to take them seriously. If we Americans can notice the adverse effects of a drug with a few years' experience, couldn't the Chinese, or any number of other cultures, notice the *beneficial* effects of an herb across centuries? Then why do our laws deny us long-used natural products just because they haven't been "proven" by an inferior method of discovering truth?

The more strictly we define our science, the less we need faith, judgment, discernment, observation, experience, wisdom, and simple common sense. These may not be scientific in the strictest sense of the word, but they are nonetheless our gifts, and in some cases, they are all we have. Perhaps our challenge is not to define a science that renders them unnecessary, but to build into our science principles that allow us to use them wisely.

9

The Elusive Properties of Wholeness

When classical scientists ask for an "account" of a relationship, or an "explanation," or the "mechanism" behind some effect, they're usually talking about what they call a "metabolic pathway." A metabolic pathway describes how chemical reactions proceed step-by-step from one to the other to achieve some purpose within the body.

For example, we know insulin has something to do with sugar. The classical scientist wants to know *exactly* what it has to do with sugar. As it turns out, insulin helps transport sugar across the cell membrane and into the cell. But even that statement isn't precise enough. To scientifically *confirm* that statement, we've got to describe the chemical structure of the molecules involved, and trace step-by-step exactly how they interact to produce the effect we're interested in. Only when we've tacked down the last detail can we conclude that we've scientifically confirmed the nature of insulin's effect in the body.

As a result, many medical research reports read more or less like this:

> We attempted to determine whether mobilization of cellular calcium or enhanced influx of extracellular Ca2+, or both, were involved in the elevation of [Ca2+]i during each of the two phases. In all experiments, the elevation of [Ca2+]i stimulated by TRH was compared with that induced by depolarization of the plasma membrane with high extracellular K+, which enhances Ca2+ influx. In medium with 1.5mM Ca2+, K+ -depolarization caused an elevation of [Ca+]i to 780 +/- 12 nM. When the concentration of Ca2+ in the medium was lowered to 0.1 mM and 0.01 mM Ca2+, peak K+ depolarization-induced elevation of [Ca2+]i was lowered to 114 +/- 3.4 and 110 +/- nM, respectively. In medium with 0.1 and 0.01 mM Ca2+, peak K+ . . . etc.

To fit natural healing therapies into that scheme of things, we must somehow express them in the same molecular terms. Consider herbs, for example. Our body breaks herbs down into specific molecules. If we're going to control how an herb enters into a metabolic pathway, we've got to do the same thing. So the first step in studying herbs scientifically is to do with them what the body does: we must break them down.

This is called "identifying and isolating the active elements," and it becomes another point of contention between conventional medicine and natural healing. Identifying and isolating the active elements *destroys* the herb. The medical principle requires it; the natural healing principle forbids it.

The Important Properties Belong to the Whole

From the natural-healing point of view, individual molecules mean nothing by themselves. Their meaning appears only as they interact within the complex makeup of the herb. The meaningful and interesting properties of the herb are those that it possesses *as a whole*, and which disappear when the herb is dismantled into its parts.

Doctors understand this sort of thing. They warn against the "interactive effects" of drugs, meaning strange and unpredictable things that happen when you mix drugs together. I mentioned earlier that chemotherapy drugs provoke cancer-like resistance in tumor cells, and that a tumor cell's resistance to *two* drugs turns out to be 100 times greater than predicted from the separate frequencies for each drug. The two drugs combined create a result you can't predict by looking at them one at a time.

Here's a more ordinary example. When Van Cliburn plays an A on the piano, he creates at least three kinds of vibrations: (1) a fundamental frequency, which makes the note an A rather than some other note on the scale; (2) certain "overtones," which make the note a *piano* A rather than, say, a clarinet A; and (3) certain vibrations of the piano case, which give the note a unique *tone quality* — a brilliance, perhaps, or a certain mellowness.

The "active element" in the mixture is probably the *fundamental frequency*, since the "A" property of the note is the one we notice most, and it's the only property that can stand alone. None of the three vibrations defines the note's *entire* function, and some of the note's most interesting properties — its "piano-ness," and its "tone quality" — don't exist anywhere except as they somehow emerge like magic when the vibrations blend together. People who accept natural healing believe the same sort of "emerging" of new properties also happens in a plant, and that we lose those new properties when we break the plant apart.

Drugs Are Neither Safer Nor More Effective Than Herbs

Advocates of conventional medicine usually argue that drugs are safer and more effective than whole herbs. They back this contention with logic, not with research. Herbs are inconsistent, they say. They contain "dozens of active ingredients in unpredictable concentrations," as one report put it, so you never know for sure what the patient is getting. Isolating lets you (a) give single substances (b) in exact amounts, so that (c) you can test *exact* effects, both positive and negative, which makes everything easier to predict and control. Hence, drugs are safer and more effective than herbs, or so they contend.

Neither research nor the logic of natural healing supports that point. The logic of natural healing says that the "dozens of active ingredients," interacting together, can serve to balance one another, enhancing good effects and reducing bad ones. An article in *Science News* magazine quotes Bruce Ames, chairman of biochemistry at the University of California at Berkeley, saying that our dietary intake of natural pesticides is "probably at least 10,000 times higher than the dietary intake of man-made pesticides." But we tend not to get cancer from them because many plants "contain natural anticarcinogens — chemicals such as Vitamins C and E, selenium and beta carotene — that neutralize the detrimental effects of the carcinogens."

I mentioned tardive dyskinesia earlier, the movement disorder caused by neuroleptic drugs that is "basically untreatable," according to *Science News*. But one treatment shows promise. It is lecithin, which, while not a whole food, is far more complex than the isolates of medicine. In one research study published in the *American Journal of Psychiatry*, researchers fed lecithin to tardive dyskinesia patients, and observed "significant improvement in the dyskinesias of all subjects during the lecithin trial, even with concomitant administration of a constant dose of neuroleptic medication."

Following the medical principle, researchers looked into lecithin to find the active ingredient. It turned out to be *choline*, which they isolated. Now they were able to compare directly the complex natural substance (lecithin) against the isolated chemical taken from it (choline). Choline was quicker — serum choline levels rose to their peak after thirty minutes versus one hour for the lecithin. But lecithin was more potent — choline produced an 86 percent increase versus a 265 percent increase for lecithin. And it was longer lasting — choline's effect disappeared after four hours, while lecithin's effect had yet to disappear after twelve hours. (The amounts taken were the same in each case.) Lecithin also showed fewer side effects.

This relative value of isolates versus wholes is currently being debated in the courts. Marijuana reduces eye pressure in glaucoma, and nausea in chemotherapy patients. But it's a "Schedule 1" drug, meaning it has "no currently accepted medical use as a treatment in the United States," and is considered unsafe even under medical supervision. So medical scientists isolated marijuana's active ingredient, THC. The Food and Drug Administration approved it as a drug in 1985. The problem, according to a *Science News* report, is that "many patients and physicians claim that purified THC is not nearly as effective as a puff of pot." Several FDA-approved studies "have demonstrated marijuana's effectiveness . . . and in some cases its advantages over THC pills." THC has side effects of its own, and a patient is quoted citing a study of THC as a drug for nausea in which "50 percent of the patients said they'd rather throw up."

I don't mean to argue in favor of marijuana, simply to point out the legal dilemma that it now poses for medicine and government regulators. There must be hundreds, perhaps even thousands, of similar cases where isolated drugs are legal, while either the herb they came from, or therapeutic claims about the herb, are not.

The Problem of Burgeoning Complexity

Albert Szent-Gyoergyi, who shared a Nobel Prize for his scientific research, died in 1986 at the age of 93. As he entered his later years, he reflected on his scientific life, which he spent pursuing nature's secrets through this process of isolation. He began by pointing out that nature creates life by combining molecules into a series of ever more complex wholes:

> At every step, more complex and subtle qualities are created, and so in the end we are faced with properties which have no parallel in the inanimate world . . . We must not lose our bearings or else we may fall victim to the simple idea that any level of organization can best be understood by pulling it to pieces, by a study of its components — that is, the study of the next lower level. This may make us dive to lower and lower levels in the hope of finding the secret of life there. This made, out of my own life, a wild goose chase.

Scientists isolated an immune system chemical that they called interferon because it seemed to interfere with cancer cells. They announced it as a "wonder drug," predicted it would cure cancer, and were surprised when it didn't. Its side effects include seizures, liver damage, and heart problems.

So they studied interferon more closely and eventually isolated three subvarieties — alpha, beta, and gamma — which they tested against cancer, separately and in combinations. Still no luck. Now they've isolated at least sixteen varieties of alpha interferon alone, and they're still hoping one or a combination of them might be the wonder drug they're looking for. If not, is the next step to subdivide the sixteen alpha varieties? And if that doesn't work, then what?

This sort of fragmenting and re-fragmenting multiplies research problems geometrically, which in turn multiplies geometrically the need for scientists and dollars. Each failure becomes a sign that we need to probe still more deeply, and the whole process eventually becomes a bit like following a path through a forest and having it branch every fifty feet or so. At some point, even the best backwoodsman has got to become confused. Perhaps this is the sort of "wild goose chase" that Albert Szent-Gyoergyi was talking about.

According to Thomas Kuhn in his *Structure of Scientific Revolutions*, such burgeoning complexity often signals that a science is approaching a "paradigm shift," or a shift in the way scientists explain things. When the old explanation meets problems it can't handle, its proponents elaborate it. When that fails, they elaborate the elaborations, until the explanation becomes *so* elaborate that it collapses under the weight of its own complexity. That may be happening to medicine today.

According to the natural healing principle, the qualities that nurture and heal are the ones that Szent-Gyoergyi sees *emerging* as nature weaves parts into wholes, then *disappearing* as we break wholes into parts. From this point of view, nature is a *creator of wholes*, "health" is the measure of wholeness, and "natural healing" is the process by which we achieve it. Isolating chemicals, which is a breaking-apart, seems not to fit.

10

What We Need Is Balance

As an example of complex and subtle qualities emerging when parts form wholes, the Chinese, who are perhaps the world's foremost proponents of natural healing, offer the *spouting bowl.*

Spouting bowls are made from bronze, with handles mounted on opposite sides of the bowl's upper rim. The "master" fills the bowl with water, then vigorously rubs the handles, which sets the bowl, and the water, vibrating. The vibrating creates waves — not ordinary waves that cross the water, but "standing waves" that go up and down. As the up-and-down motion builds, the waves merge to form a single standing wave that rises higher and higher, until it turns into a geyser-like "water spout" that may reach up to three feet high.

No one knows for sure how spouting bowls work. What western physicists have been able to discover, however, is that the spout seems to emerge from the blending of two exactly opposite waves. And *that*, more or less, symbolizes what the Chinese believe about opposites, and what we should do about them: we should balance them to form a whole that is greater than either alone can be.

Balanced Opposites Hold Each Other In Place

In America, we seem to believe that opposites ought to fight. Proponents of medicine sometimes describe those who promote natural healing with words like "fraud," "charlatan," and "huckster." Proponents of natural healing, in their turn, sometimes call medical doctors "the enemy," accuse them of "hawking" their procedures, and describe surgery as "ritual mutilation."

The Chinese would call either of those extremes "unbalanced." The Chinese virtually *exalt* balance, considering it nature's most important attribute. And they consider that the only way to achieve balance is to somehow unite opposites so that each holds the other in place.

There's a game where two people sit on the floor, facing each other, scooted close together, knees tucked against their respective chests, with the soles of their shoes touching. They extend both arms around their legs and clasp hands. Then they lean back so that they're pulling against each other's arms, and so that each person's backward lean is kept in check by the other's weight. From that position, they try to stand. The only way to do it is if each person, as they rise, exactly balances the other. If one person's weight overpowers the other, they fall over. That, more or less, is the Chinese idea of the role of balance: it keeps nature from falling over.

For example, the sun balances the implosive force of gravity against the explosive force of nuclear fusion. The planets in their orbits balance the outward thrust of centrifugal force against the inward tug of the sun's attraction. The nature and condition of *everything*, without exception, reflects the state of balance, or lack of it, achieved by the things that make it up. And the only things that can balance are opposites. Perhaps, then, when we see these opposite health paradigms, we ought not to see a call for battle, but a call for balance.

Suppose we decide to *merge* the two principles to form a single, balanced health-care system. What might that look like?

Four categories of health-related substances

To begin with, the two principles, as we discussed in earlier chapters, prefer different health-related substances. The differences, it turns out are based on (1) function, and (2) form:

- *Preferred function*: The logic of natural healing prefers substances that *nurture*; the logic of medicine prefers substances that *control*.
- *Preferred form:* The Logic of natural healing prefers *whole* substances; the logic of medicine prefers *isolated* substances.

Table 3 summarizes the differences:

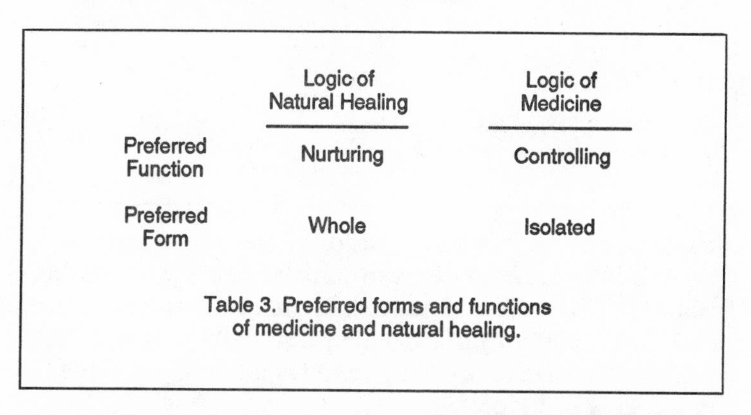

	Logic of Natural Healing	Logic of Medicine
Preferred Function	Nurturing	Controlling
Preferred Form	Whole	Isolated

Table 3. Preferred forms and functions of medicine and natural healing.

Natural healing prefers nurturing and wholeness because it considers them more *natural*. Medicine prefers controlling and isolation because it considers them more *predictable*.

When we combine the two functions and the two forms, we get four categories of health-related substances:

- Whole substances that nurture, or foods.
- Whole substances that control, or medicinal herbs.
- Isolated substances that nurture, or vitamin and mineral supplements.
- Isolated substances that control, or drugs.

Table 4 summarizes the four categories:

As you can see, foods fall in the upper-left corner of the diagram, where the two natural healing preferences intersect. Drugs fall in the lower-right corner where the two medical preferences intersect. Medicinal herbs and food

		FORM	
		Whole (Natural)	Isolated (Medical)
FUNCTION	Nurturing (Natural)	Foods, including food	Vitamin & mineral supplements
	Controlling (Medical)	Medicinal herbs	Drugs

Table 4. A four-celled diagram showing four categories of health-related substances as they relate to the preferences of the natural healing and medical princples.

supplements, in contrast, straddle the two principles, drawing one preference from natural healing, the other from medicine. What we have, then, is a *continuum*, a sort of sliding scale running from upper right to lower left, from foods to drugs, from the natural healing principle to the medical principle.

To balance the two principles, let's recognize that they apply at different times and for different purposes. Natural healing applies to health maintenance and chronic illness, where the goal is to restore the body's natural functions. Medicine, with its preference for predictability, applies to acute illness and traumatic injury, where predictability is critical, and the goal is to prevent death. The challenge in any particular case is to find the balance between the two that best suits the situation.

Table 5 represents the sliding scale from chronic to acute as it applies to the two principles, and to the four categories of health-related substances.

From this perspective, all of these health options are good *in their place*, and quackery becomes, in addition to outright deceit, any misinformed attempt by any one of these options, including medicine, to usurp the place that

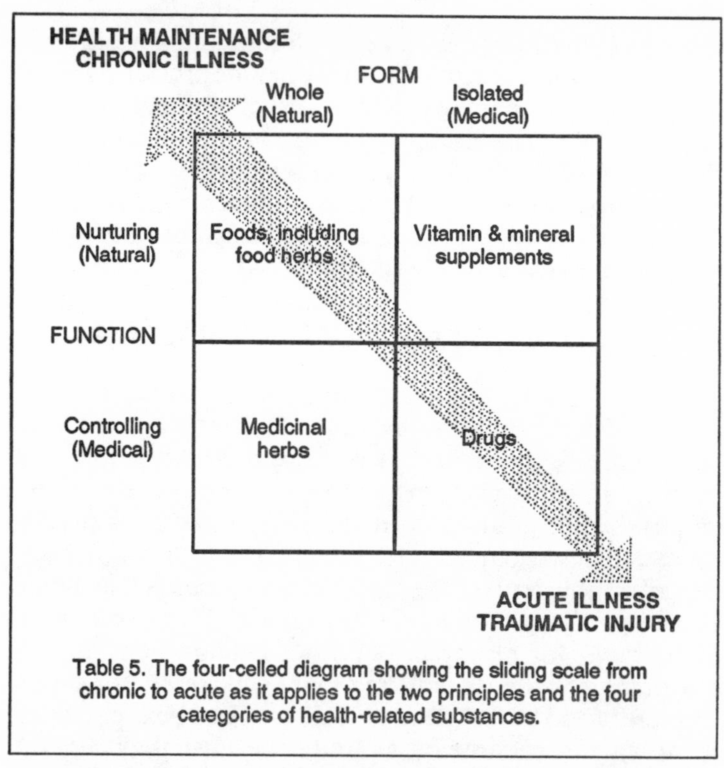

Table 5. The four-celled diagram showing the sliding scale from chronic to acute as it applies to the two principles and the four categories of health-related substances.

belongs to another, or to persuade consumers that they ought to choose a particular therapy to the exclusion of all others.

Foods and Food Supplements Apply Even During Acute Illness and Injury

Putting foods and food supplements only in the upper half of the diagram seems to suggest that nutrition can't help us during acute illnesses and accidents. That's probably when we need them most. Acute stress of any sort calls on the body to make lots of collagen, or connective tissue. But the body can't make collagen without vitamin C. According to one report, "Clinical studies provide evidence that wound healing in subjects judged not deficient in vitamin C can be significantly accelerated with supplements of this nutrient above the recommended daily allowance." Another study reported an eight-fold increase in collagen synthesis in skin cells exposed to vitamin C. A third study concluded, "Deficiencies in specific nutrients, especially proteins, vitamins, and minerals, may significantly impair the healing process. The recognition of deficits and understanding of methods of repletion are a critical part of modern surgical practice." All of this suggests that we need ample nourishment during illnesses or accidents of any sort.

Foods Are More Than Just What We Eat

When I speak of "foods," I'm referring to the view of foods as *healing substances*. According to this view, foods heal to the degree that they nurture the body's adaptive powers. To call something a "food," therefore, describes its physiological function (nurturing), and not its practical use (that we may eat it for lunch). The Chinese, in fact, describe thousands of therapeutic "food" herbs that never show up in a recipe. Some food herbs do, of course — *Dong quai*, for example, is both a healing herb, and a seasoning for the dish "Dong Quai Chicken." But other Chinese "food herbs" taste terrible (as I can bear personal witness), and become foods simply because they *heal by nurturing*, in contrast with the thousands of Chinese *medicinal* herbs that, like drugs, heal by controlling.

The problem is telling the difference — telling which herbs nurture and which herbs control. Physiologically, an herb *nurtures* if it provides raw materials for the body's adaptive processes, or if it catalyzes them, or in some way makes them more efficient. An herb *controls*, in contrast, if it interrupts or preempts the body's own control of those processes. Using that definition, our Western scientists could probably tell *analytically* which herbs nurture and which control, just by identifying the chemicals in them and figuring out how they interact with our body's chemicals. But there are tens of thousands of herbs. Analyzing them all would take forever, and so far, no one has seemed inclined to do it.

The Chinese have developed a simpler method. According to their classical philosophy, which they've been developing for at least 2,000 years, they determine whether an herb nurtures or controls by noticing its *long-*

term effects. A medicinal herb (one that controls, in other words) causes (1) *improvement*, followed by (2) a *decline*. These are the two phases of drug response that I mentioned earlier: (1) the drug's effect, and (2) the body's adaptation to it. If they notice a consistent two-phased effect from an herb, they call it "medicinal," and recommend that it be used *short term only*. Food herbs, on the other hand, have a single effect. They create improvement. Like carrots and peas, they may be used forever with no "rebound reaction," or decline. Food herbs are "kingly," or "superior." Medicinal herbs are "assistants" that occasionally supplement the kingly food herbs. This is the natural healing point of view.

I contrast this therapeutic view of nutrition with the orthodox, non-therapeutic view of nutrition that licensed dieticians practice here in the United States. Until very recently, the discipline that licenses dieticians tended to assume, like medicine, that foods *don't* heal. As a result, it concerns itself primarily with planning nourishing meals, particularly in institutions like hospitals and schools. Even today, licensed dieticians tend not to study, nor to believe in, the healing properties of foods, except, of course, for the well-documented role of vitamins and minerals in deficiency diseases like rickets and beri beri.

For this reason, I draw a careful distinction between the natural healing idea that foods may be *therapeutic* substances, and the view of orthodox medical doctors and licensed dieticians that foods are what we eat for lunch. In fact, from the natural healing perspective, foods are the *only* healing substances. Drugs do not — and *cannot* — heal, because a body that depends on outside control cannot be considered healthy.

The Diagram Covers Only Substances

You may have noticed that the four-celled diagram considers only therapeutic *substances*. From the natural healing point of view, *any* practice that strengthens the body's adaptive powers becomes therapeutic. Chiropractic thus becomes a legitimate natural healing therapy to the degree that it strengthens the body's adaptive powers by aligning the spinal column, which houses the nerves that control the organs. Color therapy, play therapy, humor therapy, breath therapy, visualizing, meditating, and so on, all become legitimate therapies to the degree that they can be demonstrated to strengthen the body's powers of adaptation, *even if they seem nonsensical*. Unlike medicine, the natural healing principle does not require scientific explanations. It requires only that something be shown to work. And it does *not* presume to judge, by logic, what makes sense and what doesn't. From the natural healing point of view, a therapy that doesn't make sense may simply mean we still have things to learn.

Homeopathy May Be a Gentle Option To Drugs

The therapy known as homeopathy doesn't fit the diagram and needs to be explained. Homeopathic remedies, like drugs, control. They do not nurture. They belong, therefore, in the bottom half of the four-celled diagram, which makes them most appropriate for acute conditions. They differ from drugs, however, in at least two important regards.

First, homeopathic remedies are designed to *worsen* symptoms, not relieve them. This sounds crazy until we remember the two-phased effect of drugs. Phase one is what the drug does to the body; phase two is how the body adapts to the drug. The two are generally opposites. Homeopathy's founder, Samuel Hahnemann, noticed this two-phased effect of drugs as early as 1792, and it prompted him to quit medicine. "Most medicines have more than one action," he wrote, "the first a *direct* action, which gradually changes into the second (which I call indirect secondary action). The latter is generally a state exactly the opposite of the former."

Hahnemann's idea was to use the *second* action to produce the healing effect. (Drugs use the first.) If the second action is to improve the patient's condition, the first action must worsen it, since the second action reverses the first. And that's why Hahnemann sought remedies that, as their first effect, would exactly mimic the patient's symptoms.

Second, Hahnemann wanted to worsen symptoms as little as possible. So he diluted his remedies, administered them, diluted them again, administered them again, and so on, always noting their effect, hoping to find the smallest possible effective dose. To his great surprise, the remedies became more powerful as they became more diluted. In fact, he got his best effect with dilutions so weak that, theoretically, not a single molecule of the therapeutic substance remained in the solution. He was healing, it seems, with pure water.

At this his medical colleagues hooted. Could he explain the effect? A spiritual principle, he said. Unscientific, they said. Test it, he said. They refused, knowing logically that it couldn't possibly work. "Is there any remedy in the Homeopathic Materia Medica that can supersede the necessity of bleeding?" one of them wrote. "Can we safely discard from our practice a remedy the success of which . . . is so firmly established every time it is judiciously used, that the prominent symptoms begin to subside the moment the blood begins to flow?"

Homeopathy currently enjoys a resurgence. Researchers have shown that dilutions beyond "Avogadro's limit" — the ones that should be pure water — affect the rotation of light in ways that pure water will not. Other researchers, using the latest Nuclear Magnetic Resonance techniques, have distinguished Hahnemann's "infinitesimal" dilutions from placebos. And recent research has shown homeopathy to be more effective than drugs alone against hay fever, arthritis, and colds.

Biological Response Modifiers Don't Strengthen the Immune System

The drugs doctors call *biological response modifiers* are supposed to strengthen the immune system, but they do it by controlling, not by nurturing, which is more or less like a father trying to *force* his son to be self-reliant. Biological response modifiers mix the *goal* of natural healing (strengthening the body's natural biological response) with the *method* of medicine (controlling).

As a result, they put doctors in the curious position of *fighting* the very immune system they hope to strengthen. For example, some biological response modifiers act as "artificial viruses." They provoke the immune system into producing more of the cells and chemicals that fight cancer. Researchers have found, however, that the body *resists* them. It produces a blood enzyme that breaks them down, and antibodies that leave them biologically inactive. So researchers made the biological response modifiers more stable, which also made them more toxic. Now they've got a version with an irregular shape that seems to confuse the body into not producing antibodies that inactivate it, and it breaks down faster, which makes it less toxic. The researchers are trying to make the immune system stronger, yet their main problem is finding some way to work around it.

One report on biological response modifiers concluded like this: "In theory, [biological response modifiers are] the perfect set up, but clinical trials have proved less than heartening . . . In many cases, [researchers] have achieved the desired immune enhancement, measured by increased interferon and NK [Natural Killer] activity. However, they have also observed toxic side effects typical of natural viral infections — fever, convulsions, and low blood pressure." In some cases, the patients died, though their deaths may have been from other factors.

After so many discouraging results, Carl Pinsky of the Sloan-Kettering Cancer Institute said, "[Even] if there's no way to change the biological responses of people with cancer . . . at least you've tested the hypothesis."

I suggest that is *not* the case — that drug research designed to control the body's immune system from the outside has *not* tested the hypothesis that the body's *own* immune response can be strengthened, since strength is measured by self-reliance, not by submission. I suggest instead that we must become willing to test natural healing's goal with natural healing's method. Until we do, we will be attacking cancer and other major diseases with a health philosophy that is, at best, barely half of a whole.

11

The Power of Personal Choice

Based on the information just presented, let's assume that natural healing and medicine form together a more complete health-care system than either forms alone, and that our challenge, when we're sick, is to choose from among the options those that will serve us best. The question now becomes, who shall do the choosing?

Here again, medicine and natural healing operate from different assumptions. William T. Jarvis, Ph.D., president of the National Council Against Health Fraud, Inc., rhetorically presented the view of conventional medicine when he asked:

> Should we license and give medicare dollars to alchemists, witches, herbalists, health food therapists, faith healers, etc., on the assumption that the consumer will be wise enough to choose the proper kind of care, and within sufficient time to protect his life and health?

Jarvis apparently doubts that we consumers are wise enough to choose for ourselves, a premise that the natural healing principle takes as an article of faith. Physicians may not doubt our wisdom when they meet us as friends, but when they accept us as *patients*, and particularly when they reach into their arsenal of tests and therapies, their training virtually *requires* that they see us as helpless and needing to be controlled. Choosing external control as a strategy, and deciding that people ought to be controlled, are two sides of the same coin.

And notice how each principle assumes about consumers exactly what it assumes about the body. The medical principle assumes that neither the body nor the consumer is wise; the natural healing principle assumes they both are, or at least they are capable of becoming so.

I see at least three arguments that favor the natural healing point of view:

Educated People Often Prefer Natural Healing

First, studies show that people who choose natural healing tend to be more educated than those who prefer medicine alone. An article in the *Annals of Internal Medicine* reported a study in which researchers from the University of Pennsylvania Cancer Center compared the education level of 304 of their Center's own medical patients and 356 patients who sought natural healing therapies that doctors consider "unproven, unorthodox or ineffective, fraudulent, and so on." Table 6 shows that people who chose natural healing tended, on the average, to be substantially more educated.

	Chose Medicine	Chose Alternatives
HS graduate only or less	62%	40%
Attended some college	18%	24%
Bachelor's degree	9%	16%
Graduate degree	11%	19%

Table 6. People who choose non-medical alternatives tend to be significantly more educated than those who choose medicine alone.

When the researchers asked why so many educated people prefer therapies that orthodox medicine calls fraudulent, they found that these people were trying to cure their cancer by *strengthening their own adaptive powers*, and medicine doesn't give them that choice. As the researchers put it, the non-medical treatments "*are geared toward improving the patient's own biologic and psychic capacity to counteract illness*. Most patients find the internal logic and global, mind-body emphasis of this perspective intuitively correct and fundamentally appealing." (Italics added.)

Contrast this with the California Medical Association's description of people who choose non-medical remedies. According to its booklet, *The Professional's Guide to Health & Nutrition Fraud*, victims of health fraud fall into four basic groups: "Unsuspecting People," "Gullible People," "Desperate People," and "Alienated People." As the *Annals of Internal Medicine* article points out, this picture simply isn't true.

(The CMA booklet describes "victims of health fraud," while I refer to "people who choose non-medical remedies." Anti-quackery advocates typically use the term "health fraud" to describe all therapies that conventional medicine doesn't approve of, with virtually no other standard of discrimination. For example, in the quote that began this chapter, National Council Against Health Fraud president William T. Jarvis [who helped prepare the CMA booklet] lumps in the same statement "alchemists, witches, herbalists, health food therapists, faith healers." In a *USA Today* article, FDA Deputy Commission John Norris defined fraudulent remedies, in essence, as anything done outside of an approved clinical setting by anyone who is not a licensed medical doctor. In reading the anti-quackery literature, you may reasonably substitute the phrase "people who choose non-medical therapies" for the phrase "victims of health fraud.")

The CMA booklet explains why "unsuspecting," "gullible, "desperate," and "alienated" people" become "victims of health fraud":

> Chronic diseases tend to be viewed by these persons not as separate disease entities, but rather as exter-

nal symptoms of an internal underlying dysfunction, disorder, or toxicity and, therefore, these patients are susceptible toward treatments *geared toward improving* their overall wellness, and strengthening *their own biological and psychic capacity to counteract illness.*

That, of course, describes the natural healing principle. Curiously, if you refer to the italicized sentence in the previous quote from the *Annals of Internal Medicine*, you'll see that the words I've italicized in the CMA quote match, virtually word for word, the logic described in the *Annals of Internal Medicine* article, which its authors describe as "intuitively correct and fundamentally appealing." Those apparently plagiarized words suggest that the authors of the California Medical Association booklet knew — even as they described "fraud" victims as "unsuspecting," "gullible," "desperate," and "alienated" — that they tend, in fact, to be more educated, on the average, than people who prefer medicine alone.

The *Annals of Internal Medicine* article also points out that 85 percent of the people who chose natural healing were using conventional medical therapies at the same time. They were apparently seeking to balance the two approaches as the last chapter recommends.

Challenges Encourage Our Wisdom To Grow

Second, medicine's assumption that we're unwise underestimates the power of *challenge* — sickness, in this instance — to call forth in us a degree of wisdom that we may not now possess. I represent this idea with the "Challenge/Wisdom Diagram." (See Figure 2)

The vertical line up the left side of Figure 2 measures the size of our challenge. The horizontal line across the bottom measures the size of our wisdom. The paired numbers (7,5) show a *level 7* challenge plotted against *level 5* wisdom. (A note to engineers: I know I've reversed the X and Y axes. It seems to work better that way.)

Now look at Figure 3. I've added a diagonal line. I call it the *Line of Mastery*, for reasons that should be obvious. The diagonal line, after all, is where the dots fall *when the*

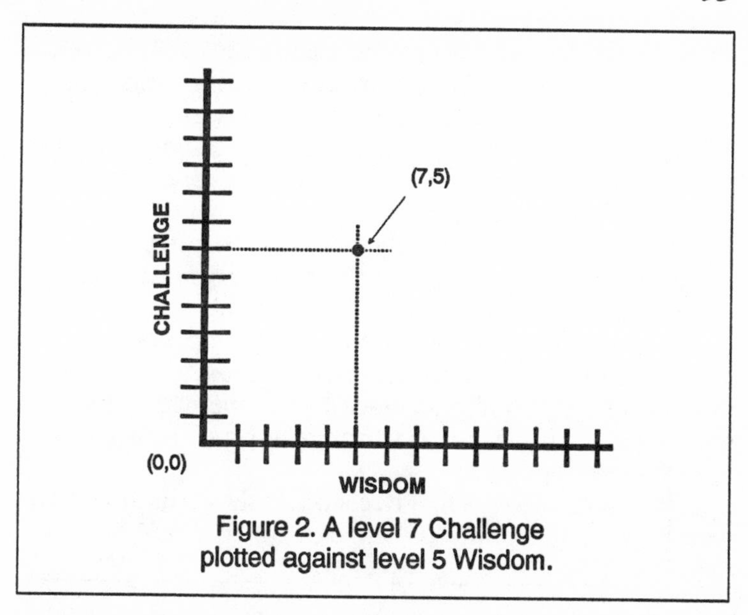

Figure 2. A level 7 Challenge plotted against level 5 Wisdom.

two numbers are equal—when our wisdom matches our challenge.

Figure 3 also plots three increasingly more trying circumstances. These could very well be illnesses. At (4,4),

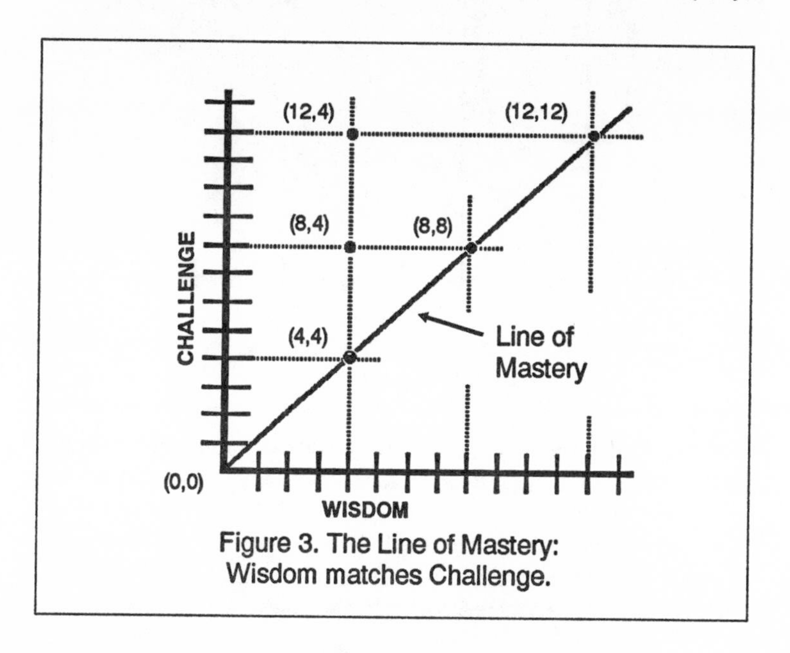

Figure 3. The Line of Mastery: Wisdom matches Challenge.

we're on the Line of Mastery; no trial there. At (8,4), we're beyond our wisdom, but probably still within coping distance. At (12,4), we're *well* beyond our wisdom, and near, or possibly beyond, the limits of what we can hope to do.

As we move from (4,4) to (12,4) and beyond, we move from knowing we can cope to not knowing. At some point, we give up. We literally stop trying to adapt, and instead cry to be rescued, or hope, at the very least, that the problem will somehow go away.

Different people have different giving-up points, and when we're challenged, each of us must decide how much trial we're willing to face before we withdraw our emotional commitment to winning and start trying merely to survive.

Figure 4 represents that decision. It shows us at (12,4), way beyond the limits of our current wisdom. We are,

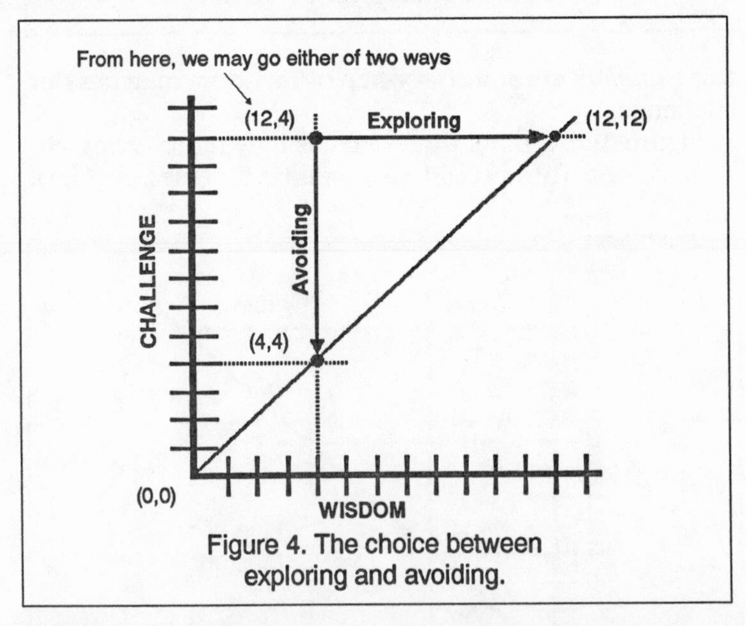

Figure 4. The choice between exploring and avoiding.

without question, *aroused*. At this point, our emotional commitment can go either of two ways: (1) we can commit to coping with the challenge, which (since we're looking for solutions) I've called *Exploring*; or (2) we can decide we can't cope, and direct our emotional energy toward getting rescued, which I've called *Avoiding*. Exploring means trying to get to (12,12); avoiding means trying to get to (4,4). On the one hand we seek to master the challenge; on the other we just want to get out of it.

What I'm suggesting is that we can't say any one of us is wise or not without taking into account whether or not we're willing to make that emotional decision. That decision *creates* wisdom, and with very few exceptions, we're all *capable* of making it, though we may choose not to risk it. Furthermore, being with people who assume we're *not* capable can *block* us from making that commitment. This is why I consider the natural healing assumption that we're capable so important. It literally calls upon us to become wise, and when we respond to that call, we *become* wise.

This is because we're governed by a principle of economy that I call the Principle of Least Effort. Basically, the Principle of Least Effort says we simply don't do what we don't have to do — physically, mentally, or emotionally. (You've seen this if you have children.) If we go to La Paz, Bolivia, where it's 12,000 feet above sea level, we'll start building new blood vessels around our heart. We don't build them here because we don't need them here. This is the Principle of Least Effort, and it applies to our adapting to sickness as well. We don't develop wisdom to overcome sickness until we get sick. And then all we have to do to get wisdom is call upon ourselves to cope. This obviously applies only to chronic illness, where the natural healing principle operates. In acute illness, we don't have time to become wise. That's why the medical principle operates there. But an acute illness can nonetheless encourage us to start getting wisdom for the next time. And whatever wisdom we get will have as its purpose to show us how to use the *natural healing* alternatives, since they alone require our wisdom.

Committing To Explore Can Help Us Heal

Third, I believe that the very effort to explore can, by itself, help us heal. I mentioned earlier the condition called "helplessness," how it creates physiological disturbances that show up in many diseases. I believe that state of helplessness is the very state of "avoiding" that the Challenge/Wisdom Diagram shows. If we just want the challenge to go away — which is what "avoiding" means — we don't call upon our inner resources, so they don't respond.

Perhaps this is why placebo responders tend to be active, responsible people. A placebo, of course, is an inactive substance that's presented as though it were a drug. Some people respond to placebos by getting better. They get fooled, in a way, so you'd expect placebo responders to be weak and gullible people. Surprisingly, the opposite turns out to be the case.

Researchers from Carnegie-Mellon University and the Rochester State Hospital studied placebo responders and found them to be (a) more men than women, (b) more women with children than women without, (c) more professional women than housewives, (d) more professional men than skilled or unskilled, (e) more educated people than uneducated, (f) more people who had experienced a traumatic interruption of their marriage than marrieds or unmarrieds, and (g) farmers — the most susceptible group of all. What these diverse groups have in common, the researchers concluded, is that "they all have heavy responsibilities, whether they want them or not." In other words, placebo responders tend to be people who have reason to *commit* to be healthy, and their bodies, we may presume, oblige them.

This growth-in-response-to-challenge principle seems to be universal. Plants grown in the still air of a greenhouse are weaker than plants grown in the challenging breezes of the out-of-doors. The bacteria that would make us sick also make us strong, just as *they* grow strong against the challenge of our antibiotics. Astronauts lose bone mass in the weightlessness of space, and regain it again back home under the challenge of gravity. A lifetime follow-up study of normal adults found that "many of the most outstanding mature adults in our entire group, many who are well-integrated, highly competent and/or creative . . . are recruited from those who were confronted with very difficult situations."

This brings us back to the question that began this debate nearly 2,500 years ago — do we, as living beings, have within us some sort of *inner adaptive power*? I would wager that we do, for what is this growth-in-response-to-challenge but *adaptation* itself? The first condition for growth is that our circumstances *require* it of us. But there is a second condition: we must also require it of ourselves.

12

Restrictive Health Laws Are Not the Answer

Sometimes, before we see an answer, we see what the answer is *not*. That seems to be the case in this instance. The answer to this challenge of balancing medicine and natural healing clearly is *not* to write laws that limit our health care choices.

Our state and national legislatures regularly consider such laws. Those who propose them generally favor medicine. They word the laws to define as "fraudulent" whatever hasn't been medically proven, which covers, of course, virtually all natural healing therapies, since the natural healing principle excludes proof of the medical sort.

Congressman Claude Pepper, for example, proposed to the 98th congress a bill (H.R. 6051) that would have established "a Strike Force on Health Quackery to coordinate the efforts of Federal agencies to curb the sale and promotion of fraudulent health remedies." The bill defined "fraudulent health remedies" as "drugs, medical devices, and medical treatment procedures which are known to be false or whose safety and effectiveness is not proven." A companion bill (H.R. 6050) proposed "criminal penalties for those who willfully sell or offer for sale drugs, devices, or medical treatment knowing that it is unsafe or ineffective or unproven for safety or efficacy."

Both bills define fraudulent practices as those that haven't been proven safe and effective, and the standards of proof are those defined by medicine, which natural healing rejects. By these bills, those who promote natural healing therapies would become criminals and subject to prosecution by a federal Strike Force. Both bills were defeated, yet the effort to pass such bills goes on.

Health Care Laws May Limit Us By Being Broad

Most anti-quackery bills make it illegal to diagnose, treat, or even attempt to prevent illness without a medical license. And they generally define words so broadly that the bills cover virtually every possible health-related substance, device, or activity. For example, the Food and Drug Administration defines a drug as anything "intended to affect the structure or any function of the body." By that definition, foods are drugs — and become subject to drug laws the instant we claim they may strengthen the body's adaptive powers. State laws often define "practice of medicine" so broadly that it literally covers a mother tending to her child's scraped knee, or neighborly inquiries about the state of someone's health. Using such laws, government regulators may bar people who don't have a medical license from virtually every aspect of practical health care.

People who believe in natural healing try to counter such laws, if they can't defeat them outright, by amending them with exceptions. They might amend a definition of drugs, for example, by adding a statement that excepts herbs, vitamin supplements, and other therapeutic foods.

People who favor medicine typically oppose these exceptions, calling them unfair, or unbalanced. In essence they say, "Why should *we* have to prove our therapies, and be licensed to use them if you don't? Everyone should meet the same standards."

I disagree. As Thomas Kuhn points out in his *Structure of Scientific Revolutions*, ways of explaining —

"paradigms" as he calls them — prescribe by their logic *their own* standards. The scientific requirement is that ways of explaining be consistent *within themselves*. Nothing in science requires that, to be fair, one must meet the standards defined by the logic of another.

Why should our laws require what science does not? Natural healing produces contextual therapies and requires the test of experience. Medicine, *by its own internal logic*, produces intrusive therapies and requires double-blind experiments. Each explanation, within itself, is consistent. Why should our laws, in the name of fairness, subject one to the requirements of the other? Each has freely and logically chosen what its therapies and its standards shall be.

Laws Shouldn't Take Sides On Scientific Issues

For that matter, why should our laws legalize explanations at all? Why should scientific issues that have yet to be resolved by scientists be *decreed* resolved by our legislatures and courts?

Even people who want to legalize medicine recognize the danger of writing scientific explanations into law, particularly when the cause is not their own. For example, The American Council on Science and Health, whose Board of Directors includes many of the most prominent names in the anti-quackery movement, recently criticized the fact that the federal government gave the Environmental Protection Agency $2.8 billion in 1987 to keep harmful chemicals out of the environment, while it gave to the National Cancer Institute only $1.2 billion for fighting cancer. Their editorial explains:

> By 1969-1970, 33 laws based on environmentalists' views were passed. Legislators had been convinced by scientific zealots predicting environmental doom . . . Congress had actually accepted and *built into the legislation* the principal assumptions of the apocalyptic movement. (Italics added.)

The problem with that sort of thing, as the editorial points out, is that it gives a legal and financial edge to people who hold certain beliefs, even as those beliefs still remain open to question. If beliefs still remain open to question, why should we enshrine them within our laws?

A Soviet Experiment In Legalizing Scientific Theory

In 1929, a young Soviet agricultural scientist named T. D. Lysenko proposed a method for increasing wheat yields. He tested his method in a single experiment on his father's farm, and it seemed to work. On the basis of that single experiment, Lysenko gained favor among Soviet bureaucrats, who were grappling with unproductive farmers and fields.

Lysenko believed in a genetic theory that the mainstream geneticists disputed. The two sides argued about both theory and policy, and the bureaucrats, who had to get about the business of growing crops, became impatient with the arguing, and decided to resolve the issue by putting Lysenko in charge.

Lysenko used his power to promote his theories. By 1948, he was able to deny money, equipment, space, and jobs to geneticists who disagreed with him. The science of genetics in the Soviet Union virtually ceased to exist.

Sixteen years later, in 1964, at a meeting of the Soviet Academy of Sciences, a young physicist named Andrei Sakharov courageously stood to protest. Referring to Lysenko's political repression of opposing scientific views, he called for an end to what he termed "infamous, painful pages in the development of Soviet science." A year later, after nearly three decades in power, Lysenko was fired.

An Imbalance of Our Own

I believe parallels exist that justify comparing the Lysenko situation to our own. Health care in America has become, by law, a privileged profession, with the privileges given to those who favor medicine, which is nothing more than a theory. Imagine one of those old-style, T-shaped scales, the kind that stands for justice. On one of the suspended plates, we stack all of the financial, political, and practical privileges given to support medicine. One the other plate we place all of the same sorts of privileges given to support natural healing. The scales don't balance. No one with the tiniest bit of sense could argue that they do. Our scales of justice favor medicine, just as the Soviet scales of justice favored Lysenkoism.

Why? What justifies the imbalance? It isn't science. If we stacked on the same scale scientific evidence for and against the two health principles, we wouldn't see the same imbalance. We'd see greater *quantities* of research on medicine, because medicine gets the research funds. But the *weight* of the evidence would *not* favor medicine. As I've tried to show in this book, the weight of scientific evidence says we need both, and that overusing medicine while underusing natural healing can make us sick.

The people who want to legalize medicine say they're doing it to protect us against fraud. To support their case, they cite stories and statistics of people who've been harmed, they say, by unproven natural healing therapies, or by being kept from the proven therapies of medicine. But laws ought to distinguish between fraud and non-fraud, not between natural healing and medicine. The two distinctions are *not* the same. We delude ourselves when we pass medical licensing laws thinking we're passing laws against fraud.

In fact, we may delude ourselves by thinking that laws can protect us against fraud in any case. This may be another instance where the cure becomes worse than the disease. Laws, like drugs, are based on the idea of external control, and subject, therefore, to the same limitations. Overused, they can only make us weak.

13

Let's Fight Fraud With Freedom

Fraud exists. But we must get rid of the notion that people are frauds just because they promote natural healing. Natural healing is neither more nor less fraudulent than medicine.

In fact, medical research is particularly susceptible to fraud because it deals, not so much with people, as with numbers, and a slight fudge of the numbers here or there can mean the difference between being published or not, or being funded or not.

Last year, the *New England Journal of Medicine* ran an article entitled "Misrepresentation and Responsibility in Medical Research." The article reviewed the work of medical researcher Robert A. Slutsky, M.D. Of the 137 articles Dr. Slutsky published in seven years, 60 were found to be either questionable or fraudulent. The fraud included "reporting numerous experiments that were never performed, reporting procedures that were incorrect or measurements that were never made, and reporting statistical analyses that were never performed."

Slutsky's fraud was detected virtually by chance. An astute reviewer read two of his articles in quick succession and noticed identical data in two supposedly independent studies. Except for that accidental good fortune, "the papers could have been read independently for years without arousing any suspicion about inaccuracy, carelessness, or fraud."

Science's alleged safeguards against fraud — peer review and replication — simply don't work. "In January 1987," the authors wrote, "a total of 752 articles were published in twenty-six of the journals in which Slutsky's articles appeared. Each of those articles, plus the articles that were rejected, required review by two or more qualified persons. Are there enough qualified reviewers," the authors ask, particularly when the research involves sophisticated techniques on the forefront of science?

The problem of too-few reviewers is compounded by the way science multiplies research problems. I mentioned earlier the case of interferon, where research has moved quickly from interferon, to three varieties of interferon — alpha, beta, and gamma — to sixteen subvarieties of alpha interferon alone. This sort of burgeoning creates what I call the "Babel effect." As the tower of knowledge grows, people end up unable talk to each other. Their language becomes confounded as each researcher pushes more deeply into the sophisticated details of his specialty, where he creates new words that only those who know what he knows have occasion to use. Each scientist stands, in a sense, on his own frontier. Where do editors go to gather a quorum of experts when no quorum exists?

The problem, the authors of the *New England Journal of Medicine* article report, is particularly acute in drug research:

> More open to abuse by fraudulent investigators are reports of symposia sponsored by pharmaceutical or instrumentation companies, since such documents are usually not peer-reviewed. Who selected the points of view in a symposium report? Who paid for its publication? Was it the subscribers (who are presumably motivated by wanting to know the results of the studies) or the drug company that wants to sell a drug to practitioners?

As for replication, I've already presented the opinion of the authors of the *New England Journal of Medicine* article: "the modern biomedical research system is structured to prevent replication — not ensure it. It appears to be impossible to obtain funding for studies that are largely duplicative."

The result of all this is that "detection [of fraud] by peer review or replication cannot be uniformly reliable . . . The emphasis on competition and the pressure to produce, while intended to advance the discovery of truth, may foster a conflict between personal career goals and the intellectual motivation of scientists to seek the truth . . . Nobody knows how frequently these conflicts occur."

". . . a conflict between personal career goals and the intellectual motivation . . . to seek the truth." That's nothing more than the old temptation to lie to become rich, famous, or powerful. Doctors succumb to it, and so do people who believe in natural healing. But believing in natural healing doesn't *incline* people to lie, any more than believing in medicine inclines people to lie. In fact, believing in natural healing ought to *prevent* lying, because the whole idea behind natural healing is that we create strength only when we honor correct principles, and that moral and ethical principles are as important as any. So the thing that leads to fraud isn't believing in natural healing, but believing we can be dishonorable and get away with it.

Meeting Fraud at its Level

That, of course, is why we have anti-fraud laws — to show frauds they can't get away with it. But laws, like drugs, only work when the dose is right. Too-loose laws encourage fraud, while too-strict laws discourage initiative and creativity. We fail on either side of a point of balance.

Our founding fathers had a good sense for this. They'd experienced two kinds of control problems. When they lived under the British, the central government had too much power. When they declared independence under the Articles of Confederation, the central government had too little power. So after the war, when they got together to write the constitution, their main question was how to distribute the power. Most of the constitutional debates focused on this very issue.

The solution our founding fathers' came up with was to give to each level of government only what the levels below it couldn't do. This principle keeps the controls as low in the government hierarchy as possible: don't write federal laws where state laws will do; don't write state laws where local laws will do; and don't write local laws where people can be taught to govern themselves.

When we violate this principle, we run into problems of what I call "scale," by which I mean the fineness of things — how big they are, how fast they move, and how much effort it takes to move them. Imagine Gulliver at a Lilliputian sock-hop and you have a good sense of "problems of scale." In hierarchical systems, higher levels always operate at slow and insensitive Gulliver-like scales, compared to the Lilliputian fineness of lower levels. The federal government is slower and clumsier than state governments; states are slower and clumsier than cities; cities are slower and clumsier than people doing things for themselves. The same principle applies to our body: the heart beats at its pace, while the chemical reactions that power it operate at an infinitely faster rhythm of their own.

We run into problems when we try to meet fast-scale challenges with slow-scale government responses. A classic example of this principle is the Rubik's Cube. Erno Rubik invented his cube in Hungary. Before long it became a world-wide craze. Rubik stood to make a fortune; Hungary had a guaranteed export bonanza.

But Hungary is a centrally planned economy. It took government committees nine months to approve the idea. Then it took another six months to order and install the manufacturing equipment. By then the craze was over. More than 100 million cubes had been sold — almost none of them Hungarian.

Consumer demand operates on one scale, central governments operate on another. The people who made the fortunes lived in free-market economies where they could decide quickly and act fast. They caught the energy of the wave because they matched its scale. Hungary didn't, and Rubik lost his cube. A Hungarian author, Mezei Andras, wrote a play about the debacle called *The Hungarian Cube*. "Everyone made money on the cube," he wrote, "except the Hungarians."

Consumer fraud, like the Rubik's Cube craze, is a fast-scale problem. Frauds don't work through bureaucracies. Those who wish to fight frauds probably shouldn't either. Frauds don't follow slow-scale rules, and when things get hot, they don't hesitate to jump from one scam to another. Honest people, on the other hand, want to build a long-term business, so they try to go along. They drop the pace of their efforts to match the slow-scale pace of the bureaucracies that regulate them and very nearly die. They try to co-exist with slow-scale regulation, while their market runs away from them at an altogether faster pace. This is how regulators put honest people out of business, while the frauds, who abuse the very foundation of the natural healing principle, skip from one scam to another and ultimately skip away.

Our only defense is to meet the problem at its level. Frauds are individual citizens trying to fool other individual citizens. That puts the problem at the lowest and fastest possible scale, meaning we really have no choice but to expect people to handle this one virtually on their own. What we ought to be looking for are ways to sharpen each citizen's ability to discern.

Forbidden Information

Discerning obviously takes information. It's interesting to note, therefore, that one effect of our current health-care laws is to block the flow of information.

I can sell just about any health product I want, as long as I don't tell you what it's supposed to do, or why I think it will work. To give you that information, I've got to get it approved by the Food and Drug Administration, which approves virtually nothing but medical research.

Even some medical research doesn't get approved. For example, I mentioned earlier the study by Ewan Cameron and Linus Pauling that showed vitamin C working against cancer. Here are findings from other research on vitamin C and the immune system:

- Vitamin C corrected a defect in immune system cells' ability to move in response to a chemical signal.
- It improved the migration and "phagocytosis" (cell-eating ability) of immune system cells.

- It increased the responsiveness of T cells.
- It enhanced the production and effect of interferon, a critical immune system chemical.
- It amplified the production of antibodies, which destroy invading cells.
- It protected against anaphylactic shock, a potentially fatal immune system overreaction.
- It inhibited the effect of certain carcinogens.
- It enhanced the encapsulation and isolation of tumors by connective tissue.

All of these finding appear in medical literature, yet no manufacturer or seller may mention them in connection with a vitamin C product.

Sometimes research itself gets blocked. I mentioned earlier a study of Chinese herbs conducted at the University of Texas. A report of the study published in the journal *Cancer* presented these results:

> This communication describes a remarkable augmentative effect *in vitro* by two Chinese medicinal herbs on T cell function . . . The extract from *astragalus membranaceous* [one of the herbs] induced a restored function in nine of ten patients . . . The extract from *ligustrum lucidum* likewise effected an immune restoration in nine of 13 cancer patients . . . This degree of immune restoration appears to be complete . . . since [it] approximates or even exceeds the [immune reaction] observed among normal healthy control subjects. Such complete restoration was not observed with the more conventional well-defined drugs such as indomethacin or cimetidine.

The quote says, in essence, that a test-tube study of cancer cells showed the herbs up to 90 percent effective in restoring complete immunity against cancer, even to the point that it exceeded the level of immunity in normal, healthy cells. The report also stated that "preliminary clinical trials with herbs (in China) indicated that they could augment nonspecific cellular immune responses in cancer patients after a course of treatment *in vivo*."

A *Los Angeles Times* report of the study stated that the herbs:

- protected cancer patients against the damaging effects of chemotherapy and radiation.
- prolonged life in patients with liver cancer.
- may prolong life in the elderly by removing from the blood those T-suppressor cells that make them more vulnerable to diseases of all types as they multiply in old age.
- may help AIDS patients rebuild their immunity.

Intrigued by these reports, I called the project's director, only to learn that his funds for the research had been cancelled, and his laboratory space reduced. He's given up and gone on to other things, not because the research lacked promise, but because it lacked political support. I offered to find private funds for the research, and he declined, explaining that, unless the research was approved through normal channels, going on with it could only cause him trouble — an example of the imbalanced scales of privilege that I spoke of earlier.

Suppose I decide to continue the research myself. I could sell the herbs without more research, but I wouldn't be able to say anything about them. So I decide to apply for FDA approval. According to the statistics, I should expect to spend about $70 million per product, after which (assuming I succeed, which is unlikely) I will be able to both sell my herbs *and* advertise what they do.

But so will everybody else. I can't patent those herbs, so I have no claim on them. Other people can use my FDA approval to market and advertise the herbs without having to recover my development costs. So I'm forced to charge more than my competitors, they capture my market, and I go out of business.

Protection From What Helps Us

The net effect of our current laws is to set up a filter that passes only certain kinds of information about health products and therapies. Studies of drugs pass the filter; studies of herbs and nutrients don't. Double-blind studies pass; correlational studies don't. Test tube studies pass; clinical studies don't.

Nor does information about traditional remedies. Researchers discovered those Chinese anti-cancer herbs in centuries-old Chinese medical classics. We tend to discount such sources, calling them "unscientific." Yet those herbs appear to work, which probably shouldn't surprise us. After all, is experience more likely to preserve what helps, or what harms or has no value? *Science 82* magazine published an article about ancient Indians in Peru who surveyed canals down steep mountain slopes at such precise angles, and following such sophisticated scientific principles, that we would have to use satellites and laser beams to match them. *Science News* magazine reported that certain North American Indians planted crops along the top of curiously shaped mounds that apparently raised the temperature several degrees and gave the Indians a week or two extra growing time in the fall. Why should traditional cultures be any less discerning about their health?

Foreign research also tends not to pass the filter, despite FDA claims to the contrary. In a *U.S. News and World Report* article, FDA Deputy Commissioner John Norris complains that trying to enforce antiquackery laws is "like holding back the tide." The article warns us that "countless cures without a shred of value lure patients away from legitimate treatments that could save lives," and cites as its main example a natural healing product that's widely used in European hospitals, and favorably reviewed in more than 200 European research studies. Is it truly "without a shred of value"? Or is it simply foreign to our way of thinking?

Proponents claim these restrictions protect us against fraud. Yet they don't restrict fraud; they restrict correlational studies, studies of herbs and nutrients, clinical studies, information about traditional remedies, and foreign research. By what logic are we better off "protected" from these things? It's true we can read them in books, but not as they apply to particular products, which is when we need them most.

Let the Principles Find Their Place

Suppose the laws were loosened. Suppose those who wish to serve us were allowed to support their claims with those now-prohibited forms of knowledge that come from experience rather than experiment. And suppose the laws governing health-care practices were changed to keep a measure of quality-control, yet allow natural healing therapists as much right to practice as physicians? Would fraud increase?

I doubt it. If the amount of fraud did increase, however, so would the amount of truth, since the current laws restrict them both. And since quality tends to survive in an open marketplace, I would wager that the net effect of freedom would be an overall increase in truth. And health.

We, of course, would be required to discern. But what of it? We're required to discern anyway. And since the current laws restrict information, we'd probably discern more clearly if we had information to do it with.

And in our discerning, we would have to come to grips with the conflict between natural healing and conventional medicine. This would be open competition now, with no privileged position granted to one or the other. Which would win? My guess would be neither. And both. Because winning isn't the point. The point is to be free to choose, and to have information to choose with. From freedom, I predict, would come balance, with each of the principles settling into its place — natural healing for chronic illness and general health, with medicine reserved for those acute and traumatic conditions where it truly saves lives.

Appendix

A List of Natural Healing Resources

To compile the following list, we called organizations we knew were involved in natural healing, and asked them to refer us to others with similar interests. A number of them referred us to directories compiled by themselves or others, which we reviewed. The organizations and publications we've listed here came from those sources. Some are medically oriented, yet apparently open to natural healing alternatives, which supports the balanced approach we recommend in the book. While we've tried to select those that appear to have gained a measure of respect and support within the industry, we endorse none of them, nor do we vouch for their expertise or credibility. We offer this list to you as a place to begin your inquiries should you desire to further pursue any aspect of natural healing. Please use judgment and discernment in dealing with the natural healing industry as you would with any other.

FOUNDATIONS AND ASSOCIATIONS

AL-ANON
(Information for relatives
and friends of alcoholics)
P.O. Box 182
Madison Square Station
New York, NY 10010
(212)473-6200

ALCOHOLICS ANONYMOUS
P.O. Box 459
Grand Central Station
New York, NY 10017
(212)473-6200

ALLIANCE FOR ALTERNATIVE MEDICINE
P.O. Box 59
Liberty Lake, WN 99019
(509)255-9246

ALS SOCIETY OF AMERICA
15300 Ventura Blvd., Suite 315
Sherman Oaks, CA 91403
(818)340-7500

ALZHEIMER'S DISEASE AND RELATED DISORDERS ASSOCIATION
360 N. Michigan Ave., Suite 1102
Chicago, IL 60601
(312)864-0045

AMERICAN ANOREXIA NERVOSA ASSOCIATION, INC.
133 Cedar Lane
Teaneck, NJ 07666
(201)836-1800

AMERICAN ASSOCIATION FOR RELIGIOUS THERAPISTS
7175 SW 45th St.
Ft. Lauderdale, FL 33314
(305)475-8489

AMERICAN ASSOCIATION OF BIOFEEDBACK CLINICIANS
2424 Dempster
Des Plaines, IL 60016
(312)827-0440

AMERICAN ASSOCIATION OF NATUROPATHIC PHYSICIANS
P.O. Box 33046
Portland, OR 97233
(503)255-4863

AMERICAN BOARD OF PREVENTIVE MEDICINE
Department of Community Medicine
Wright State University
P.O. Box 927
Dayton, OH 45401
(513)278-6915

AMERICAN CHIROPRACTIC ASSOCIATION
1916 Wilson Blvd.
Arlington, VA 22201
(703)276-8800

AMERICAN COLLEGE OF ADVANCEMENT IN MEDICINE
23121 Verdugo Dr.
Laguna Hills, CA 92653
(714)583-7666

AMERICAN HOLISTIC MEDICAL ASSOCIATION
2002 Eastlake Ave. E
Seattle, WA 98102
(206)322-6842

AMERICAN INSTITUTE OF STRESS
124 Park Ave.
Yonkers, NY 10703
(914)963-1200

AMERICAN LONGEVITY ASSOCIATION
1000 W. Carson St.
Torrance, CA 90509
(213)544-7057

AMERICAN NAPRAPATHIC ASSOCIATION
5913 W. Montrose Ave.
Chicago, IL 60634
(312)282-2686

AMERICAN OSTEOPATHIC ASSOCIATION
212 E. Ohio St.
Chicago, IL 60611
(312)280-5800

AMERICAN SCHIZOPHRENIA ASSOCIATION
Huxley Institute for Biosocial Research
900 N. Federal Highway
Boca Raton, FL 33064
(407)393-6167

AMERICAN TINNITUS ASSOCIATION
P.O. Box 5
Portland, OR 97207
(503)248-9985

ANAD
(National Association of Anorexia Nervosa
and Associated Disorders)
P.O. Box 271
Highland Park, IL 60035
(312)8313438

CALIFORNIA COALITION FOR HEALTH RIGHTS
333 S. Indian Ave., Suite E
Palm Springs, CA 92262
(619)327-2199

CANCER CONTROL SOCIETY
2043 N. Berendo St.
Los Angeles, CA 90027
(213)663-7801

CENTER FOR SCIENCE IN THE PUBLIC INTEREST
1501 16th St., N.W.
Washington, D.C. 20036
(202)332-9110

CENTER FOR THE STUDY OF ANOREXIA AND BULIMIA
1 West 91st St.
New York, NY 10024
(212)595-3449

CITIZENS COMMISSION ON HUMAN RIGHTS
P.O. Box 41837
Sacremento, CA 95841
(916)988-6334

FEINGOLD ASSOCIATION OF THE U.S.
(Behavior disorders)
P.O. Box 6550
Alexandria, VA 22306
(703)768-3287

FOUNDATION FOR INNOVATION IN MEDICINE
411 North Ave. E
Cranford, NJ 07016
(201)272-2967

GINSENG RESEARCH INSTITUTE
P.O. Box 42
Roxbury, NY 12474
(607)326-4843

HERB RESEARCH FOUNDATION
1780 55th St.
Boulder, CO 80301
(303)449-2265

HIPPOCRATES HEALTH INSTITUTE
25 Exeter St.
Boston, MA 02116
(617)523-6525

HOLISTIC HEALTH ASSOCIATION
360 Nassau St.
Princeton, NJ 08540
(609)924-8580

HUMAN ECOLOGY RESEARCH FOUNDATION/SW
8345 Walnut Hill Ln.
Dallas, TX 75231
(214)361-9515

HUXLEY INSTITUTE
900 N. Federal Highway, Suite 330
Boca Raton, FL 33432
(407)393-6167

INSTITUTE FOR CHILD BEHAVIOR RESEARCH
4182 Adams Ave.
San Diego, CA 92116
(619)281-7165

INTERNATIONAL ACADEMY OF NUTRITION AND PREVENTIVE MEDICINE
P.O. Box 5832
Lincoln, NE 68505
(402)467-2716

INTERNATIONAL ACADEMY OF
HOLISTIC HEALTH & MEDICINE
218 Avenue B
Redondo Beach, CA 90277
(213)540-0564

INTERNATIONAL ASSOCIATION OF CANCER VICTORS AND FRIENDS
7740 W. Manchester
Playa del Ray, CA 90293
(213)822-5032

INTERNATIONAL ASSOCIATION OF CLINICAL NUTRITIONISTS
P.O. Box 5832
Lincoln, NB 68505
(402)467-2716

INTERNATIONAL CHIROPRACTORS ASSOCIATION
1901 L St., N.W.
Washington, D.C. 20036
(202)659-6476

INTERNATIONAL FOUNDATION FOR HOMEOPATHY
2366 Eastlake Ave. E, Suite 301
Seattle, WA 98102
(206)324-8230

LA LECHE LEAGUE INTERNATIONAL, INC.
9616 Minneapolis Ave.
Franklin Park, IL 60131
(312)455-7730

MANDALA HOLISTIC HEALTH
P.O. Box 1233
Del Mar, CA 92014
(619)481-7751

NATIONAL CENTER FOR HOMEOPATHY
1500 Massachusetts Ave., N.W.
Washington, D.C. 20005
(202)223-6182

NATIONAL HEALTH FEDERATION
P.O. Box 688
Monrovia, CA 91016
(818)357-2181

NATIONAL WOMEN'S HEALTH NETWORK
1325 "G" Street, N.W.
Washington, D.C. 20005
(202)347-1140

NATURAL FOOD ASSOCIATES
P.O. Box 210
Atlanta, TX 75551
(214)796-3612

NORTHWEST INSTITUTE OF ACUPUNCTURE AND ORIENTAL MEDICINE
1141 NW Market Street
Seattle, WA 98107
(206)789-1399 (Clinic), (206)789-1290 (School)

NUTRITION EDUCATION ASSOCIATION
3647 Glen Haven
Houston, TX 77025
(713)665-2946

NUTRITION FOR OPTIMAL HEALTH
ASSOCIATION
P.O. Box 380
Winnetka, IL 60093
(312)835-5030

NUTRITION SOCIETY OF AMERICA
500 Dorian Rd.
Westfield, NJ 07090
(201)233-4788

PEOPLE'S MEDICAL SOCIETY
14 E. Minor St.
Emmaus, PA 18049
(215)967-2136

PRICE-POTTENGER NUTRITION
FOUNDATION
5871 El Cahone Blvd.
San Diego, CA
(619)582-4168

READ NATURAL CHILDBIRTH
FOUNDATION
P.O. Box 956
San Rafael, CA 94915
(415)456-8462

SEATTLE MIDWIFERY SCHOOL
2524 16th Street
Seattle, WA 98144
(206)322-8834

THE STROKE FOUNDATION, INC.
898 Park Ave.
New York, NY 10021
(212)734-3461
TOURETTE SYNDROME ASSOCIATION
41-02 Bell Blvd.
Bayside, NY 11361
(718)224-2999

PUBLICATIONS

ANTI-AGING
Box 1067
Hollywood, FL 33022
BETTER NUTRITION
390 Fifth Ave.
New York, NY 10018
BIO-PROBE NEWSLETTER
4401 Real Ct.
Orlando, FL 32808
JEFFREY BLAND'S PREVENTIVE MEDICINE UPDATE
3215 56th St.
Gig Harbor, WA 98355
CANCER NEWS JOURNAL
International Association of Cancer Victors and Friends
7740 Manchester #110
Playa del Rey, CA 90203
CHOICE
Committee for Freedom of Choice in Medicine
146 Main St., #408
Los Altos, CA 94022
COMPLEMENTARY MEDICINE
J.S.B. and Associates
3215 56th St., N.W.
Gig Harbor, WA 98335
DOCTORS DATA NEWSLETTER
Box 111
West Chicago, IL 60185

FEELING BETTER!
P.O. Box 58036
Tierra Verde, FL 33715

HEALTH CONSCIOUSNESS
Roy Kupsinei, M.D.
Box 550
Oviedo, FL 32765

HEALTH FACTS
Center for Medical Consumers
237 Thompson St.
New York, NY 10012

HEALTH FREEDOM NEWS
Box 688
Monrovia, CA 91016

HEALTH PLUS PUBLISHERS
P.O. Box 22001
Phoenix, AZ 85028

HEALING CURRENTS:
Trends in the Art of Health
Tapestry Communications
P.O. Box 529
Springville, UT 84663

HERALD OF HOLISTIC HEALTH NEWSLETTER
1766 Cumberland Green, Suite 208
St. Charles, IL 60174

HERB BUSINESS BULLETIN
PO Box 32
Berryville, AR 72616

HOLISTIC LIFE
2223 El Cajon Blvd., #426
San Diego, CA 92104

HOLISTIC MEDICINE
American Holistic Medical Association
3932 Little River Tpk
Annandale, VA 22003

INTERNATIONAL JOURNAL OF HOLISTIC HEALTH AND MEDICINE
P.O. Box 955
Mill Valley, CA 94942

MEDICAL HOTLINE
119 W. 57th St.
New York, NY 10019

NATURAL FOOD AND FARMING
P.O. Box 332
Atlanta, TX 75558
NEW TEXAS MAGAZINE
4314 Medical Parkway
Austin, TX 78756
PEOPLE'S DOCTOR NEWSLETTER
P.O. Box 982
Evanton, IL 60204
PEOPLE'S MEDICAL SOCIETY
NEWSLETTER
14 Minor St.
Emmaus, PA 18049
PREVENTION
Rodale Press
33 E. Minor St.
Emmaus, PA 18049
PUBLIC CITIZEN HEALTH RESEARCH GROUP
(Magazines, newspapers, booklets)
2000 P St., N.W.
Washington, D.C. 20036
PURE FACTS
(Newsletter of the Feingold
Association of the U.S.)
P.O. Box 6550
Alexandria, VA 22306
T'AI CHI CH'UAN NEWSLETTER
Wayfarer Publications
P.O. Box 26156
Los Angeles, CA 90026
TODAY'S LIVING
390 5th Ave.
New York, NY 10018
TOWNSEND LETTER FOR DOCTORS
911 Tyler St.
Port Townsend, WA 98368
WHOLISTIC LIVING NEWS
Association for Holistic Living
P.O. Box 16346
San Diego, CA 92116

SCHOOLS

ACUPRESSURE WORKSHOP
1533 Shattuck Ave.
Berkeley, CA 94709
(415)845-1059

ACUPUNCTURE EDUCATION CENTER
R.D. #1, Box 7A Muhlig Rd.
Parksville, NY 12768
(914)428-8833

AMERICAN COLLEGE OF NUTRIPATHY
6821 E. Thomas Rd.
Scottsdale, AZ 85251
(602)946-5515

AMERICAN SCHOOL OF DRUGLESS THERAPY
P.O. Box 101
Highland Heights, KY 41076
(606)441-2644

ANTIOCH UNIVERSITY
650 Pine St.
San Francisco, CA 94108
(415)956-1688

BIOFEEDBACK SOCIETY OF AMERICA
4301 Owens St.
Wheat Ridge, CO 80033
(303)422-8436

CALIFORNIA ACUPUNCTURE ASSOCIATION
1922 Westwood Blvd.
Westwood, CA 90025
(213)390-7911

CALIFORNIA SCHOOL OF HERBAL STUDIES
P.O. Box 39
Forestville, CA 95436
(707)887-7457

CENTER FOR CHINESE MEDICINE
230 S. Garfield Ave.
Monterey Park, CA 91754
(213)721-0774

CHICAGO NATIONAL COLLEGE OF NAPRAPATHY
3330 N. Milwaukee Ave.
Chicago, IL 60641
(312)282-2686

LIFE SCIENCE INSTITUTE
6600-D Burleson Rd.
Austin, TX 78744
(512)385-2781

CREATIVE HEALTH INSTITUTE
918 Union City Rd.
Union City, MI 49094
(517)278-6260

INTERNATIONAL INSTITUTE OF REFLEXOLOGY
P.O. Box 12642
St. Petersburg, FL 33733
(813)343-4811

JOHN BASTYR COLLEGE OF NATUROPATHIC MEDICINE
1408 N.E. 45th St.
Seattle, WA 98015
(206)632-0354

JOHN F. KENNEDY UNIVERSITY
12 Altarinda Rd.
Orinda, CA 94563
(415)254-0200

MATERNITY CENTER
119 E. San Antonio Ave.
El Paso, TX 79901
(915)778-9815

MIDWEST CENTER FOR STUDY OF ORIENTAL MEDICINE
1222 W. Grace St.
Chicago, IL 60613
(312)975-1295

MYOTHERAPY SCHOOL OF UTAH
3018 E. 3300 S., P.O. Box 9036
Salt Lake City, UT 84109
(801)484-1912

NATIONAL CENTER FOR HOMEOPATHY
1500 Massachusetts Ave., N.W., #163
Washington, DC 20005
(202)223-6182

NATIONAL COLLEGE OF NATUROPATHIC MEDICINE
11231 S.E. Market St.
Portland, OR 97216
(503)255-4860

NATIONAL HOLISTIC INSTITUTE
5299 College Ave.
Oakland, CA 94618
(415)547-6442

NATIONAL INSTITUTE FOR
NUTRITIONAL EDUCATION
5600 Greenwood Plaza Blvd., Suite 205
Greenwood Village, CO 80111
(303)771-7951

THE NATURAL GOURMET COOKERY SCHOOL
48 West 21st St., 2nd Floor
New York, NY 10010
(212)645-5170

NUTRITIONISTS INSTITUTE OF AMERICA
312 W. 8th St.
Kansas City MO 64105
(816)842-2942

RYOKAN COLLEGE
1258 Venice Blvd.
Mar Vista, CA 90066
(213)390-7560

SCHOOL OF NATURAL HEALING
P.O. Box 412
Springville, UT 84663

OHASHI INSTITUTE
52 W. 55TH St.
New York, NY 10019
(212)684-4190

TRADITIONAL ACUPUNCTURE
INSTITUTE
American City Bldg., #108
Columbia, MD 21044
(301)596-6006

VERMONT COLLEGE
Box 70
Montpelier, VT 05602
(802)485-2000

Notes & References

Introduction

Page

1 *84-year-old man*: de la Monte, S.M. et al. "Fatal Disseminated Bacillus Calmette-guerin Infection and Arrested Growth of Cutaneous Malignant Melanoma Following Intralesional Immunotherapy." *American Journal of Dermatopathology* 8 (August 1986) p. 331-335.

Chapter 1
Beware the Whoops! Factor

Page

7 *Buzzards*: Some time ago I ran across this quote and wrote it down, but I didn't record the source, nor have I been able to find it. I decided to use the quote anyway because it adds a touch of interest without affecting my arguments. If you happen to know the source, please let me know so I can add it to future editions.

8 *Moldboard plow:* "The Disappearing Land."

Newsweek (August 22, 1982) p. 24-28. • *Alcoholic detoxification centers*: "Vagrants Pack Units to 'Dry Out'." UPI wire story appearing in *The* [Provo, Utah] *Daily Herald* (August 22, 1982) p. 54. • *Landfills*: "Are Landfills A Major Threat to Climate?" *Science News* 131 (March 7, 1987) p. 150. • *Minority businesses*: Blake, D. "Are Set-Aside Programs Helping Anybody?" *D&B Reports* 35 (July/August 1987) p. 38-39.

9 *$25 billion*: The approximate $25 billion figure for cancer research expenditures since 1971 came by summing and averaging figures presented in *National Cancer Program: Director's Report and Annual Plan* for several representative years. The report is published yearly by the National Institutes of Health. • *Chemotherapy*: Schimke, R.T. "Methotrexate Resistance and Gene Amplification." *Cancer* 57 (May 1986) p. 1912-1917. • *Bacteria*: "Bacteria". *The World Book Encyclopedia*. Chicago: World Book, Inc., 1988, vol. 2, p. 19-22. • *Chicken feed*: "Animal Drug Feeds: The Human Threat." *Science News* 110 (September 18, 1976) p. 183.

10 *Gene amplification*: For gene amplification as a mechanism of cancer resistance, see Schimke, R.T. "Methotrexate Resistance and Gene Amplification." *Cancer* 57 (May 1986) p. 1912-1917. For gene amplification as a resistance mechanism in bacteria, see Hornemann, U. et al. "Spectinomycin Resistance and Associated Dna Amplification in Streptomyces Achromogenes Subsp. Rubradiris." *Journal of Bacteriology* 169 (June 1987) p. 2360-2366. • *Heidigger*: Heidigger's views are described in Prigogine, I. and Stengers, I. *Order Out of Chaos: Man's New Dialogue with Nature*. New York: Bantam Books, 1984, p. 33. The quotes come from the authors' description of Heidigger's views, rather than from Heidigger himself.

11 *Prigogine*: Prigogine, I. and Stengers, I. *Order Out• of Chaos: Man's New Dialogue with Nature*. New York: Bantam Books, 1984, p. 21. •

Weinberg: Weinberg, R. A. "The Molecules of Life." In *The Molecules of Life: Readings from Scientific American.* New York: W.H. Freeman and Company, 1985, p. 1-11.

Chapter 2
Medicine Takes Healing From Nature's Hands

Page

13 *Rush*: Coulter, H. *Divided Legacy: A History of the Schism in Medical Thought*. Richmond, CA: North Atlantic Books, 1973, vol. 3, p. 53-54.

15 *Misadministered drugs*: Brand, D.A. et al. "Adequacy of Antitetanus Prophylaxis in Six Hospital Emergency Rooms." *New England Journal of Medicine* 309 (September 15, 1983) p. 636-640. • *Nicked arteries*: Orcutt, M.B. et al. "Iatrogenic Vascular Injury. A Reducible Problem." *Archives of Surgery* 120 (March 1985) p. 384-384. • *Phlebitis*: Falchuk, K.H. et al. "Microparticulate-induced Phlebitis. Its Prevention by In-line Filtration. *New England Journal of Medicine 312 (January 10, 1985) p. 78-82.* • *Infections from other patients*: See note on "Iatrogenic deaths" below. • *Infants hospitalized with fevers*: DeAngelis, C. et al. "Iatrogenic Risks and Financial Costs of Hospitalizing Febrile Infants." *American Journal of Disease of Children* 137 (December 1983) p. 1146-1149.

16 *Pediatric group practice*: Kramer, M.S. et al. "Adverse Drug Reactions in General Pediatric Outpatients." *Journal of Pediatrics* 106 (February 1985) p. 305-310. • *Wrong test results*: Asper, R. et al. "Critical Aspects of Urine and Stone Analysis." *Urologia Internationalis* 41 (1986) p. 334-342. • *Colon cancer*: Schipper, H. et al. "Carcinoma of the Colon Arising at Ureteral Implant Sites Despite Early External Diversion: Pathogenetic and Clinical Implications." *Cancer* 47 (April 15, 1981) p. 2062-2065. • *36% of 815 patients*: Steel, K. et al. "Iatrogenic Illness on a General Medical Service at a University Hospital."

New England Journal of Medicine 304 (March 12, 1981) p. 638-642. • *Intensive care unit*: Trunet, P. et al. "The Role of Iatrogenic Disease in Admissions to Intensive Care." *Journal of the American Medical Association* 244 (December 12, 1980) p. 2617-2620. • *Iatrogenic deaths*: The Centers for Disease Control researcher who helped me calculate the figure of 700,000 deaths was Teresa Horan. She also shared with me figures from a major study that showed 5.5% of hospital patients become infected from other patients. These are called "nosocomial infections." The study also showed that nosocomial infections kill 20,000 people per year, and contribute to the death of another 60,000. • The study showing a death rate from treatment-caused illnesses of .05 percent is cited in "The Sickly Side of Hospital Stays." *Insight* (April 18, 1988) p. 48-49. The figure comes from the Medical Insurance Feasibility Study, sponsored by the California Medical Association and the California Hospital Association. Copies of the full report are available from Sutter Publications, Inc, 731 Market Street, San Francisco, CA 94103.

19 *Bi-phasic effect of drugs*: Kosten, T.R. et al. "A Preliminary Study of Beta Endorphin During Chronic Naltrexone Maintenance Treatment in Ex-opiate Addicts." *Life Sciences* 39 (July 7. 1986) p. 55-59. Also Tortella, F.C. et al. "Electroencephalographic and Behavioral Effects of D-ala2-methionine-enkephalinamide and Morphine in the Rat." *Journal of Pharmacology and Experimental Therapeutics* 206 (September 1978) p. 636-643; Takahashi, L.K. et al. "Intracranial Sites Regulating the Biphasic Action of Progesterone in Estrogen-primed Golden Hamsters." *Endocrinology* 119 (December 1986) p. 2744-2754. And Thayer, R.E. "Energy, Tiredness, and Tension Effects of a Sugar Snack Versus Moderate Exercise." *Journal of Personality and Social Psychology* 52 (January 1987) p. 119-125. (This last study doesn't show direct physiological

changes, but it shows a two-phased behavioral effect of taking sugar, which has drug-like properties in that it can stimulate endorphin activities. "The sugar snack condition was associated with significantly higher tension after 1 hr, and a pattern of initially increased energy and reduced tiredness, followed 1 hr later by increased tiredness and reduced energy.") Also, Judith Hooker and Dick Teresi, in *The 3-Pound Universe* (New York: Macmillan Publishing Company, 1986, p. 76), report the initial euphoria over L-dopa as a treatment for Parkinson's disease, and the disillusionment that followed:

> L-dopa was not an undiluted magic potion, however. After a brief halcyon period, it typically unleashed a new chamber of horrors — grotesque hallucinations, delirium, murderous furies, compulsive growling, gnashing of teeth, involuntary movements, delusions, tics, compulsive cursing, to name just a few of the "side effects." [Neurologist Oliver] Sacks tells of patients seesawing erratically between two pathological poles — the rigid, withdrawn "imploded" state of Parkinsonism and an "exploded" psychotic state. Moral? To Sacks it is the "utter inadequacy of mechanical medicine, the utter inadequacy of a mechanical world view." As we shall see, the brain is not a simple machine that can be repaired by adding X grams of a single chemical.

Anabolic steroids: Lamb, D.R. "Anabolic Steroids in Athletics: How Well Do They Work and How Dangerous Are They?" *American Journal of Sports Medicine,* (January-February 1984) p. 31-38. • *Endorphin blockers and SIDS*: Orlowski, J.P. "Cerebrospinal Fluid Endorphins and the Infant Apnea Syndrome." *Pediatrics* 78 (August 1986) p. 233-237.

20 *Endorphin increase in mice*: Rosecrans, J.A. et

al. "Biphasic Effects of Chronic Nicotine Treatment on Hypothalamic Immunoreactive Beta-endorphin in the Mouse." *Pharmacology, Biochemistry and Behavior* 23 (July 1985) p. 141-143. • *Same thing happening in humans*: Baranowska, B. et al. "The Role of endogenous opiates in the Mechanism of Inhibited Luteinizing Hormone (LH) Secretion in Women with Anorexia Nervosa: The Effect of Naloxone on LH, Follicle-stimulating Hormone, Prolactin, and Beta-endorphin Secretion." *Journal of Clinical Endocrinology and Metabolism* 59 (September 1984) p. 412-416.

21 *Blood-brain barrier*: The techniques for crossing the blood-brain barrier is described in "Complex Courier Delivers Dopamine," *Science News* 123 (April 16, 1983) p. 249. • *Schimke*: Schimke, R.T. "Methotrexate Resistance and Gene Amplification." *Cancer* 57 (May 1986) p. 1912-1917. • *"aim is to prevent resistance"*: Silberner, J. "Resisting Cancer Chemotherapy," *Science News* 131 (January 3, 1987) p. 12-13. Also, "In the past years, scientists have discovered many of the obstacles — including drugs, radiation, and natural immune defenses — that metastatic cells can overcome . . . If, as the evidence now shows, metastases arise from cancer cells that are the ultimate survival artists, continually evolving, then they form a constantly moving target against which conventional weaponry is doomed . . . The usual method is to use as much radiation and drugs as possible and then, when resistance develops, substitute another drug or combination. But because of what we know about the nature of cancer and the way it spreads, that may not make much sense. The drugs and X rays used to kill cancer cells, [cancer specialist Joshua] Fidler says, may kill or exhaust cells necessary to defense and thus allow more rapid proliferation of metastatic cells." (Rodgers J.A. "Catching Cancer Strays." *Science 83*, July/August 1983, p. 46, 48. • *"inhibit the inhibitor"*: "Sear-

ching for the Better Clot-buster," *Science News* 133 (April 9, 1988) p. 230.

Chapter 3
Medicine Confronts The Second Law

Page

23 *Second Law and genetic processes:* All of the physiological principles presented in this chapter are described in Doolittle, R.F. "Proteins". In *The Molecules of Life: Readings from Scientific American*. New York: W.H. Freeman and Company, 1985.

30 *Rush*: Coulter, H. *Divided Legacy: A History of the Schism in Medical Thought*. Richmond, CA: North Atlantic Books, 1973, vol. 3, p. 53-54. • *"its own greatest protector"*: Reuter, F. "Folk remedies and human belief systems." *The Skeptical Inquirer* 11 (Fall 1986) p. 48.

Chapter 4
An Ancient Principle Reasserts Itself

Page

33 *Hippocrates*: Castiglioni, A. *A History of Medicine.* New York: Alfred A. Knopf, 1958, p. 172. • Democritus: Edwards, P. *Encyclopedia of Philosophy*. New York: The Free Press, 1967, vol. 1, p. 193-198.

34 *Galen*: Brock, A.J. *Greek Medicine.* New York: J. M. Dent & Sons, 1929, p. 152. • 1800-page history: Coulter, H. *Divided Legacy: A History of the Schism in Medical Thought.* Volumes 1 and 2 are published by the Weehawken Book Company, Washington, D.C., 1975 and 1977. Volume 3, is published by North Atlantic Books, Richmond California, 1982. • "an inspiring idea": Edwards, P. *Encyclopedia of Philosophy.* New York: The Free Press, 1967, vol. 1, p. 195. • "dethroned": Edwards, P. *Encyclopedia of Philosophy.* New York: The Free Press, 1967, vol. 4,

see the entry under "Hippocrates."

36 *Taxonomy of diseases*: Hudson, R.P. *Disease and Its Control*. Westport, Connecticut: Greenwood Press, 1983, p. 236. • Taken from *Tree structure*: *Medical Subject Headings - Tree Structures*. 1988. Bethesda, Maryland: National Library of Medicine, 1988.

37 *CMA booklet*: Taken from *The Professional's Guide to Health and Nutrition Fraud*. San Francisco: California Medical Association, (undated).

38 *Two forms of imbalance in the immune system*: For an easy-to-understand explanation of the immune system that confirms the points made here, see Mizel, S. B. and Jaret, P. *The Human Immune System: The New Frontier in Medicine*. New York: Simon & Schuster, Inc., 1985.

40 *Fluxes*: Prigogine, I. and Stengers, I. *Order Out of Chaos: Man's New Dialogue with Nature*. New York: Bantam Books, 1984, p. 127.

41 *Billfolds*: "Good News and Social Behavior." *Science News* 110 (December 18 & 25, 1976) p. 395. • *Optimism and health*: Peterson, C. et al. "Explanatory Style and Illness." *Journal of Personality* 55 (June 1987) p. 237-265.

42 *Concentration of potassium*: Szent-Gyoergyi, A. "Drive in Living Matter to Perfect Itself." *Journal of Individual Psychology* 22 (November 1966) p. 153-162.

Chapter 5
Two Briefs in the Case Against Cancer

Page

43 *Conventional medical theory*: Schimke, R.T. "Methotrexate Resistance and Gene Amplification." *Cancer* 57 (May 1986) p. 1912-1917. • *Cancer as a process*: Weinstein, I.B. "Cell Culture Studies on the Mechanism of Action of Chemical Carcinogens and Tumor Promoters. *Carcinogenesis: A Comprehensive Survey* 10 (1985) p. 177-187.

44 *Cancer cells suffer mutations no more often*

than normal cells: Rubin, H. "Cancer as a Dynamic Developmental Disorder." *Cancer Research* 45 (July 1985) p. 2935.• *Gene amplication as cancer process*: See Weinstein article cited immediately above. Also Cillo, C.D. et al. "Generation of Drug-resistant Variants in Metastatic B16 Mouse Melanoma Cell Lines." *Cancer Research* 47 (May 1987) p. 2604-2608. Stark, G.R. "DNA Amplification in Drug Resistant Cells and in Tumours." *Cancer Surveys* 5 (1986) p. 1-23. Slaga, T.M. et al. "Cellular and biochemical changes during multistage skin tumor promotion." *International Symposium of the Princess Takamatsu Cancer Research Fund* 14 (1983) p. 291-301. Hayashi, K. et al. "Increase in Frequency of Appearance of Cadmium-resistant cells Induced by Various Tumor Promoters: Evidence for the Induction of Gene Amplification." *International Symposium of the Princess Takamatsu Cancer Research Fund* 14 (1983) p. 255-259. • *Schimke quote*: Schimke, R.T. "Methotrexate Resistance and Gene Amplification." *Cancer* 57 (May 1986) p. 1912-1917. • *Another expert*: Stark, G.R. "DNA Amplification in Drug Resistant Cells and in Tumours." *Cancer Surveys* 5 (1986) p. 1-23. • *Resistance to high doses of toxic metals*: Koropatnick, J. et al. "Acute Treatment of Mice with Cadmium Salts Results in Amplification of the Metallothionein-1 Gene in Liver." *Nucleic Acids Research* 13 (August 12, 1985) p. 5423-5439. • *Gene amplification in response to repeated small toxic doses, but not single large dose*: Schimke, R.T. "Methotrexate Resistance and Gene Amplification." *Cancer* 57 (May 1986) p. 1912. • *"Genes amplify at a precise moment*: Kellems, R.E. et al. "Amplified Dihydrofolate Reductase Genes Are Located in Chromosome Regions Containing DNA that Replicates During the First Half of S-phase." *Journal of Cell Biology* 92 (February 1982) p. 531-539. • *Human growth hormone and five other proteins*: Choo, K.H. et al. "Cosmid Vectors for High Efficiency DNA-mediated Transformation and Gene Amplification in Mammalian Cells: Studies with the Human Growth Hormone Gene." *Gene* 46 (1986) p. 277-286. Also, Schimke, R.T. "Methotrexate Resistance and Gene Amplification." *Cancer* 57 (May 1986) p. 1913. • *Insulin and interferon encourage gene amplification*: Kellems, R.E. et al. "Amplified Dihydrofolate Reductase Genes are located in Chromosome Regions Containing DNA that Replicates During the First Half of S-phase." *Journal of Cell Biology* 92 (February 1982) p. 531-539. Also, Barsoum, J. et al. "Mitogenic Hormones and Tumor Promoters Greatly Increase the Incidence of Colony Forming Cells Bearing Amplified Dihydrofolate Reductase Genes." *Proceedings of the National Academy of the Unites States* 80 (September 1980) p. 5330-5334. And, Morris, S. et al. "Transient Response of Amplified Metallothionein Genes in CHO Cells to Induction by Alpha Interferon." *Molecular and Cellular Biology* 7 (June 1987) p. 600-605. • *Genes exposed to one toxin may develop resistance to unrelated toxins at the same time*: Scotto, K. W. et al. "Amplification and Expression of Genes Associated with Multidrug Resistance in Mammalian Cells." *Science* 232 (May 9, 1986) p. 751-755. • *Genes amplification is temporary at first, then can become permanent*: Rubin, H. "Cancer as a Dynamic Developmental Disorder." *Cancer Research* 45 (July 1985) p. 2939. And Snapka, R.M. et al. "Loss of Unstably Amplified Dihydrofolate Reductase Genes from Mouse Cells is Greatly Accelerated by Hydroxyurea." *Proceedings of the National Academy of Sciences of the United States* 80 (December 1980) p. 7533-7537.

45 *Gene amplification is how bacteria come to resist antibiotics*: Hornemann, U. et al. "Spectinomycin Resistance and Associated DNA Amplification in Streptomyces Achromogenes Subsp. Rubradiris." *Journal of Bacteriology* 169

(June 1987) p. 2360-2366. • *Cells take order from their context*: For a complete discussion of the idea that embryo cells take their order from their context (including the "lizard tail" example and the example of the kidney cells that developed "prostatic activity"), see Rubin, H. "Cancer as a Dynamic Developmental Disorder." *Cancer Research* 45 (July 1985) p. 2939. Also Tsonis, P.A. "Embryogenesis and Carcinogenesis: Order and Disorder." *Anticancer Research* 7 (1985) p. 617-624.

46 *Electric fields as context*: Rubin, H. "Cancer as a Dynamic Developmental Disorder." *Cancer Research* 45 (July 1985) p. 2939. • *Cells pass soluble chemicals to one another*: Robertson, M. "Nerves, Molecules and Embryos." *Nature* 278 (April 26, 1979) p. 778-780. • *Timing of cell cycles*: See the Robertson reference immediately above.

47 *When scientists culture cells in a dish*: For a discussion of all of the information presented in the section "Cells lose control in a weak context," see Rubin, H. "Cancer as a Dynamic Developmental Disorder." *Cancer Research* 45 (July 1985) p. 2939.

48 *Cartilage cells "quickly lose their capacity," and "Cells . . . will lose their malignant character"*: Both quotes come from Rubin, H. "Cancer as a Dynamic Developmental Disorder." *Cancer Research* 45 (July 1985) p. 2939.

49 *Gene amplification as mechanism by which cells resist chemotherapy*: Schimke, R.T. "Methotrexate Resistance and Gene Amplification." *Cancer* 57 (May 1986) p. 1912-1917. • *250- to 350-fold amplification*: Maurer, B.J. et al. "Novel Submicroscopic Extrachromosomal Elements Containing Amplified Genes in Human Cells." *Nature* 327 (June 1987) p. 434-437. • *Chemotherapy "dramatically" increased gene amplification*: See the research cited in Schimke, R.T. "Methotrexate Resistance and Gene Amplification." *Cancer* 57 (May 1986) p. 1913.

The word "dramatically" is Schimke's own. • *Effect of combining drugs*: Schimke, R.T. "Methotrexate Resistance and Gene Amplification." *Cancer* 57 (May 1986) p. 1912-1917. • *"Stimulates tumor viability"*: Levina, N.V. "Chromosomes and Drug Resistance of Tumors." *Eksperimentalnaia Onkologiia* 6 (1984) p. 14-19. • *"Growth advantage"*: Stark, G.R. "DNA Amplification in Drug Resistant Cells and in Tumours." *Cancer Surveys* 5 (1986) p. 1-23. • *"shortened survival"*: Johnson, B.E. et al. "myc Family Oncogene Amplification in Tumor Cell Lines Established from Small Cell Lung Cancer Patients and its Relationship to clinical status and Course." *Journal of Clinical Investigation* 79 (June 1987) p. 1629-1634. • *"Convert benign tumors to more lethal form"*: Schimke, R.T. "Methotrexate Resistance and Gene Amplification." *Cancer* 57 (May 1986) p. 1915.

50 *"on a plateau"*: Silberner, J. "Resisting Cancer Chemotherapy." *Science News* 131 (January 3, 1987) p. 13. • *"doses of drugs should be sufficient . . . to result in cell death"*: Schimke, R.T. "Methotrexate resistance and gene amplification." *Cancer* 57 (May 1986) p. 1915. • *Reduced binding affinity*: Haber, D.A. et al. "Properties of an Altered Dihydrofolate Reductase Encoded by Amplified Genes in Cultured Mouse Fibroblasts." *Journal of Biological Chemistry* 256 (September 1981) p. 9501-9510. • *Altered transport*: Sirotnak, F.M. et al. "Relative Frequency and Kinetic Properties of Transport Defective Phenotypes Among Methotrexate-resistant L1210 Cell Lines Derived *in vivo*." *Cancer Research* 41 (November 1981) p. 4447-4452.

Chapter 6
Medicine and the Context of Helplessness

Page

54 *Inescapable stress*: Laudenslager, M. L. et al. "Coping and Immunosuppression: Inescapable

but not Escapable Shock Suppresses Lymphocyte Proliferation." *Science* 221 (August 5, 1983) p. 568-570. • *Several kinds of chemicals become disturbed*: Drugan, R.C. et al. "Opioid and Non-opioid Forms of Stress-induced Analgesia: Some Environmental Determinants and Characteristics." *Behavioral and Neural Biology* 35 (July 1982) p. 251-264. MacLennan, A. J. et al. "Corticosterone: A Critical Factor in an Opioid Form of Stress-induced Analgesia." *Science* 215 (March 19, 1982) p. 1530-1532. • *The immune system weakens*: Laudenslager, M. L. et al. "Coping and Immunosuppression: Inescapable but not Escapable Shock Suppresses Lymphocyte Proliferation." *Science* 221 (August 5, 1983) p. 568-570. • *Cancer*: Shavit, Y. "Stress, Opioid Peptides, the Immune System, and Cancer." *Journal of Immunology* 135 (August 1985) p. 834s-837s. • *Diabetes*: Gibson, M.J. et al. "Streptozotocin-induced Diabetes is Associated with Reduced Immunoreactive beta-endorphin Concentrations in Neurointermediate Pituitary Lobe and with Disrupted Circadian Periodicity of Plasma Corticosterone Levels." *Neuroendocrinology* 41 (July 1985) p. 64-71. • *High blood pressure*: de Jong, W. et al. "Role of Opioid Peptides in Brain Mechanisms Regulating Blood Pressure." *Chest* 83 (February 1983) p. 306-308. • *Arthritis*: Millan, M.J. et al. "A model of Chronic Pain in the Rat: Functional Correlates of Alterations in the Activity of Opioid Systems." *Journal of Neuroscience* 7 (January 1987) p. 77-87. • *PMS:* Giannini, A.J. et al. "Hyperphagia in Premenstrual Tension Syndrome." *Journal of Clinical Psychiatry* 46 (October 1985) p. 436-438. • *Alzheimer's disease*: Jolkkonen, J.T. et al. "beta-Endorphin-like Immunoreactivity in Cerebrospinal Fluid of Patients with Alzheimer's Disease and Parkinson's Disease." *Journal of the Neurological Sciences* 77 (February 1987) p. 153-359. • *Depression*: Cohen, M.R. et al. "Plasma Cortisol and beta-endorphin Immunoreactivity in

Nonmajor and Major Depression." *American Journal of Psychiatry* 141 (May 1984) p. 628-632. • *Anorexia*: Yim, G.K. et al. "Opioids, Feeding, and Anorexia." *Federation Proceedings* 43 (November 1984) p. 2893-2897. • *Bulimia*: Fullerton, D.T. et al. "Plasma Immunoreactive beta-endorphin in Bulimics." *Psychologie Medicale* 16 (February 1986) p. 59-63. • *Autism*: Sahley, T.L. et al. "Brain Opioids and Autism: An Updated Analysis of Possible Linkages." *Journal of Autism and Developmental Disorders* 17 (June 1987) p. 201-216. • *Schizophrenia*: Beal, M.F. et al. "Effects of Neuroleptic Drugs on Brain beta-endorphin Immunoreactivity." *Neuroscience Letters* 53 (January 21, 1985) p. 173-178. • *Epilepsy*: Olson, G.A. et al. "Endogenous Opiates: 1983." *Peptides* 5 (1984) p. 984. • *Uncontrollability as a key element in the physiology of helplessness*: Laudenslager, M. L. et al. "Coping and Immunosuppression: Inescapable but not Escapable Shock Suppresses Lymphocyte Proliferation." *Science* 221 (August 5, 1983) p. 568-570.

55 *Overcoming a connective tissue disease*: Cousins, N, *Anatomy of an Illness*. New York: Bantam Books, 1981; *Treadmill test*: Cousins, N. *The Healing Heart*. New York: Norton, 1983.

56 *Cameron/Pauling study*: Cameron, E. and Pauling, L. "Supplemental Ascorbate in the Supportive Treatment of Cancer: Prolongation of Survival Times in Human Cancer." *Proceedings of the National Academy of Sciences of the United States of America* 73 (October 1976) p. 3685-3689. • *Double-blind study*: Creagan, E.T. et al. "Failure of High-dose Vitamin C (Ascorbic Acid) Therapy to Benefit Patients with Advanced Cancer. A controlled trial." *New England Journal of Medicine* 301 (September 27, 1979) p. 687-690. (Note: The authors of this study say patients in both groups survived a median of "about seven weeks." Jack Z. Yetiv, M.D., Ph.D., in his book *Popular Nutritional Practices* [New York:

Dell Publishing, 1986, p. 205] summarizes the study and reports a median survival of 51 days for both groups. I've used Yetiv's figures in my table. Also, Cameron and Pauling report mean figures, while Creagan and his colleagues use medians. I report both sets of figures as "averages," which isn't statistically precise, but seemed to me the best I could do under the circumstances.)

57 *Three stages of adaptation to stress*: Selye, H. *The Stress of Life* (rev. ed). New York: McGraw-Hill Book Co., 1976, p. 163. •

58 *Vitamin C in the production of corticoid hormones*: See Douglas, N.L. et al. "Effect of Ascorbic Acid on Guinea Pig Adrenal Adenylate Cyclase Activity and Plasma Cortisol." *Journal of Nutrition* 117 (June 1987) p. 1108-1114. Also, Odumosu, A, "Ascorbic Acid and Cortisol Metabolism in Hypovitaminosis C Guinea Pigs." *International Journal for Vitamin and Nutrition Research* 52 (1982) 176-185. And Liakakos, D. et al. "Inhibitory Effect of Ascorbic Acid (Vitamin C) on Cortisol Secretion Following Adrenal Stimulation in Children." *Clinica Chimica Acta* 65 (December 15, 1975) p. 251-255. • *Vitamin C in the immune response*: See Fraser, R.C. et al. "The Effect of Variations in Vitamin C Intake on the Cellular Immune Response in Guinea Pigs." *American Journal of Clinical Nutrition* 33 (April 1980) p. 839-847. Also, Anderson, R. et al. "The Effects of Increasing Weekly Doses of Ascorbate on Certain Cellular and Humoral Immune Functions in Normal Volunteers." *American Journal of Clinical Nutrition* 33 (January 1980) p. 71-76. And Anthony, H.M. et al. "Severe Hypovitaminosis C in Lung-cancer Patients: The Utilization of Vitamin C in Surgical Repair and Lymphocyte-related Host Resistance." *British Journal of Cancer* 46 (September 1982) p. 354-367. The Anthony study also showed that most cancer patients have vitamin C levels "below the thresholds for incipient clinical scurvy," and that

"levels were diet-dependent and could be increased by oral supplements." The article concluded, "Vitamin C is necessary for phagocytosis and for the expression of cell-mediated immunity." Epidemiological studies have also shown that populations of cancer patients typically have low-vitamin C diets compared to healthy populations. (See Graham, S, "Dietary Factors in the Epidemiology of Cancer of the Larynx." *American Journal of Epidemiology* 113 (June 1981) p. 675-680. Also Kolonel L.N. et al. "Role of Diet in Cancer Incidence in Hawaii." *Cancer Research* 43 (May 1983) p. 2397s-2402s). And vitamin C inhibited skin tumors in hairless mice exposed to ultraviolet light. (See Dunham, WB, "Effects of Intake of L-ascorbic Acid on the Incidence of Dermal Neoplasms Induced in Mice by Ultraviolet Light." *Proceedings of the National Academy of Sciences of the United States of America* 79 (October 1976) p. 3685-3689.)

59 *Terminal cancer patients in Selye's Stage of Exhaustion*: A number of studies show elevated corticoid levels in cancer victims. (See Feldman, J.M. et al. "Urinary Free Cortisol Excretion in Patients with Metastatic Cancer." *American Journal of the Medical Sciences* 278 (September-October 1979) p. 149-152; Also Schaur, R.J. et al. "Tumor Host Relations. II. Influence of Tumor Extent and Tumor Site on Plasma Cortisol of Patients with Malignant Diseases." *Journal of Cancer Research and Clinical Oncology* 93 (April 12, 1979) p. 287-292.) • *Increases in cortisol production of cancer patients within six months before death*: Lichter, I. et al. "Serial Measurement of Plasma Cortisol in Lung Cancer." *Thorax* 130 (February 1975) p. 91-94. • *Direct links between cortisol and the course of cancer*: Uspenskaia, L.P. et al. "Cortisol Content in the Blood Plasma in Lung Cancer." *Voprosy Onkologii* 24 (1978) p. 58-61.

60 *Decreased immunity in medical students*: Glaser, R. et al. "Stress-related Impairments in

Cellular Immunity." *Psychiatry Research* 16 (November 1985) p. 233-239. • *Physiological effects of anticipating stress*: Bychkov, V.P. et al. "Dietary Prevention of Certain Changes in the Human Body in the Presence of Neuro-emotional Stress." *Kosmicheskaia Biologiia I Aviakosmicheskaia Meditsina* 13 (September/October 1979) p. 19-22.

61 Kuhn, T. *The Structure of Scientific Revolutions*, 2d ed. Chicago: University of Chicago Press, 1970. See in particular chapter III, "The nature of normal science."

Chapter 7
The Perils of Double-blindness

Page

63 *Adverse drug reactions in a pediatric clinic*: Kramer, M.S. et al. "Adverse Drug Reactions in General Pediatric Outpatients." *Journal of Pediatrics* 106 (February 1985) p. 305-310. • *Tardive dyskinesia*: "TD Hazards Among the Retarded." *Science News* 129 (April 19, 1986) p. 248. See also "Frog Defense: Make Snakes Yawn." *Science News* 132 (October 3, 1987) p. 215. • *Using drugs for things they haven't been tested for*: See the first *Science News* reference on this page. Other evidence exists that doctors may, at times, take less care with drugs than they might. For example, "The typical physician spends three minutes on insomnia complaints and then prescribes sleeping pills without investigating the causes . . . What's more, these pills lose their effectiveness if used continually for two weeks. In fact, if they are used for months on end, which is common among chronic insomniacs, they are physically addictive and can actually cause severe sleep disturbances rather than counter them." ("The Science of Sleep." *Science News* 115 [March 26, 1977] p. 204.) Also, concerning reports that use of "estrogens and progesterones during pregnancy could lead to

cardiovascular defects in offspring": "How much scientific evidence is necessary to convince physicians of the dangers of prescribing such hormones during pregnancy remains to be seen. In January 1975, the Food and Drug Administration warned physicians against prescribing progesterones for pregnancy testing and to prevent threatened miscarriage. However, the Health Research Group, a consumer organization in Washington, reported on the basis of drug industry records that in the year following the FDA's warning, doctors wrote 500,000 hormone prescriptions for pregnant women, the same as before the warning." ("Female Hormones and Birth Defects," *Science News* 115 [January 22, 1977] p. 54-55.)

65 *Toxicity and effect vary with time of day*: Hrushesky W.J. "Circadian Timing of Cancer Chemotherapy." *Science* 228 (April 1985) p. 73-75. Also, Olson G.A. et al. "Endogenous Opiates: 1983." *Peptides* 5 (1984) p. 986. This review article reports the following: "Even the lethal dose of morphine in mice varies greatly with circadian rhythms, morphine being three to four times more potent at midnight than at 8 a.m." • *Diurnal cycles vary with age*: Reinberg, A. et al. "Aspects of Chronopharmacology and Chronotherapy in children. *Chronobiologia* 14 (July-September 1987) p. 303-325. • *Foods alter effects of drugs*: "'That foods can influence the metabolism of a drug is important,' the researchers conclude in the Dec. 3 SCIENCE, 'because changes in an individual's diet or differences between the diets of different individuals can contribute, respectively, to intraindividual and interindividual variability in the bioavailability and, consequently, in the biological effect of the drug.'" ("Steak, Diet and Drug Metabolism." *Science News* 114 (December 11, 1976) p. 376.)

66 *"Vigorous compensatory activation" of the blood pressure system*: Cody, R.J. et al. "Renin System Activity as a Determinant of Response to

Treatment in Hypertension and Heart Failure." *Hypertension* 5 (September-October 1983) p. 36-42 • *Amplifying genes*: Schimke, R.T. "Methotrexate Resistance and Gene Amplification." *Cancer* 57 (May 1986) p. 1912-1917. • *Changes become permanent*: Rubin, H. "Cancer as a Dynamic Developmental Disorder." *Cancer Research* 45 (July 1985) p. 2939.

67 *Intelligence*: Partridge, E. *Origins: A Short Etymological Dictionary of Modern English*, 4th ed. New York: Macmillan Publishing Co., Inc., 1966, p. 345-346.

Chapter 8
Experience Is the Better Test

Page

69 *"derogatory"*: Engelhardt T.H. "The Concepts of Health and Disease." In Engelhardt, H.T. Jr. and Spicker, S.F. (eds.), *Evaluation and Explanation in the Biomedical Sciences*. Dordrect, Holland: D. Reidel Publishing Company, 1975, p. 132. • *"demonic activity"*: King, L.S. "Explanations of Disease: Historian's viewpoint." In Engelhardt, H.T. Jr. and Spicker, S.F. (eds.), *Evaluation and Explanation in the Biomedical Sciences*. Dordrect, Holland: D. Reidel Publishing Company, 1975, p. 22.

70 *Chiropractic*: Jarvis W.T. "Chiropractic: A Skeptical View," *The Skeptical Inquirer* 12 (Fall 1987) p. 47.

71 *Acupuncture*: Cited in Schwartz, R. "Acupuncture and Expertise: A Challenge to Physician Control." *The Hastings Center Report* 11 (April 1981) p. 7. The person cited is Dr. George Ulett, *Journal of the American Medical Association*, February 20, 1981, p. 721. • *Chinese herbs*: "Chinese Derive Cancer Treatments from Ancient Herbal Tonics, Common Plants." *The Los Angeles Times*, October 6, 1983, part I-B, p. 5. • *"smoke screen"*: West, S. "Behind a Smoke Screen."*Science 84*, May 1984, p. 12. R. J. Reynolds ads appear in *Time* magazine on

February 6, 1984; March 19, 1984; April 30, 1984, and May 14, 1984.

73 *Replication as a "myth"*: The quote comes from Engler, R.L. et al. "Misrepresentation and Responsibility in Medical Research." *The New England Journal of Medicine* 317 (November 26, 1987) p. 1383-1389.

Chapter 9
The Elusive Properties of Wholeness

Page

75 *Metabolic pathways*: This pursuit of metabolic pathways has led scientists to develop techniques so precise that they can observe molecular movements to within just a few billionths of a meter. For example, using an enhanced version of a technique called *differential interference contrast microscopy*, scientists have observed an enzyme called kinesin as it carries materials along a microtubule that runs from a cells' interior to its rim ("Tracking a Molecule's Progress." *Science News* 133 [February 13, 1988] p. 103). Although scientists develop these techniques and obviously intend to use them, many instances exist where scientists accept explanations that haven't been confirmed so precisely. However, scientists commonly demand a stricter-than-normal standard of scientific proof when the issue is controversial. The problem in this particular controversial issue is that demand for strict proof is so one-sided. Anti-quackery advocates call natural therapies unscientific because no one can say exactly how they work, despite the fact that many medical therapies would be unscientific by the same standard. And they often cite stories of people harmed by herbs, yet condemn similar stories as unscientific, or "anecdotal evidence," when advocates of natural healing present them as evidence of an herb's benefits. • *Insulin*: Guyton, A.C. *Function of the Human Body*. Philadelphia: W.B. Saunders Company,

1974, p. 427.

76 *"mobilization of cellular calcium" quote*: Gershengorn, M.C. et al. "Thyrotropin-releasing Hormone (TRH) Stimulates Biphasic Elevation of Cytoplasmic Free Calcium in GH3 cells. Further Evidence that TRH Mobilizes Cellular and Extracellular Ca2+." *Endocrinology* 116 (July 1985) p. 217-25.

77 *Two chemotherapy drugs*: Schimke, R.T. "Methotrexate Resistance and Gene Amplification." *Cancer* 57 (May 1986) p. 1914. • *"dozens of active ingredients"*: "Take Two Puffs and Call Me in the Morning: Proponents of Marijuana's Medical Benefits Take Their Case to Court." *Science News* 133 (February 20, 1988) p. 122-123.

78 *"10,000 times"*: "Cancer and Cuisine." *Science News* 124 (October 1, 1983) p. 217. • *Basically untreatable*: "Frog Defense: Make Snakes Yawn." *Science News* 132 (October 3, 1987) p. 215. • *"significant improvement"*: Jackson, I.V. et al. "Treatment of Tardive Dyskinesia with Lecithin." *American Journal of Psychiatry* 136 (November 1979) p. 1458-1460. • *Choline vs. Lecithin:* Wurtman, R.J. et al. "Lecithin Consumption Raises Serum-free Choline Levels." *Lancet* 8028 (July 9, 1977) p. 68-69. And Gelenberg, A.J. et al. "Choline and Lecithin in the Treatment of Tardive Dyskinesia: Preliminary Results from a Pilot Study." *American Journal of Psychiatry* 136 (June 1979) p. 772-776. • *Marijuana*: "Take Two Puffs and Call Me in the Morning: Proponents of Marijuana's Medical Benefits Take Their Case to Court." *Science News* 133 (February 20, 1988) p. 122-123.

79 *"wild goose chase"*: Szent-Gyoergyi, A. "Drive in Living Matter to Perfect Itself." *Journal of Individual Psychology* 22 (November 1966) p. 153-162.

80 *Interferon*: Mizel, S.B. and Jaret, P. *The Human Immune System: The New Frontier in Medicine*. New York: Simon & Schuster, Inc., 1985, p. 88. Also, "'With interferon, we learned a lesson,' says

Hillton Levy, head of the molecular virology section of the National Institute of Allergy and infectious Disease (NIAID) at the Frederick (Md.) Cancer Research Facility. 'We thought it would be the wonder drug and were shocked when it wasn't . . . Part of the problem with interferon injections, Levy says, is that mixtures of alpha, beta and gamma interferons are probably necessary for the substance to have any effect in a given disease or tumor state. 'There are 16 different types of alpha interferon alone,' he says, 'each of which has different biological activity.' The tricky part is knowing which particular interferons are needed for which diseases." (Bennett, D.W. "Drugs that Fight Cancer...Naturally." *Science News* 128 (July 1985, p. 58.) • ***Paradigm shift***: Kuhn, T. *The Structure of Scientific Revolutions*. 2d ed. Chicago: University of Chicago Press, 1970. See in particular chapter VII, "Crisis and the emergence of scientific theories."

Chapter 10
What We Need is Balance

Page

81 *Spouting bowls*: Temple, R. *The Genius of China*. New York: Simon & Schuster, 1986, p. 41.

85 *Wound healing accelerated by vitamin C*: Ringsdorf, W.M. et al. "Vitamin C and Human Wound Healing." *Oral Surgery, Oral Medicine, Oral Pathology* 53 (Mar 1982) p. 231-236.

86 *Eight-fold increase*: Murad, S. et al. "Regulation of Collagen Synthesis by Ascorbic Acid." *Proceedings of the National Academy of Sciences of the United States* 78 (May 1981) p. 2879-2882. • *Deficiencies may impair the healing process*: Ruberg, R.L. "Role of Nutrition in Wound Healing." *Surgical Clinics of North America* 64 (Aug 1984) p. 705-714. • *Foods as healing substances:* See references immediately above. Also, "Diet can have a dramatic influence on the prevention and treatment of cancer. Spontaneous regression of cancers, for instance, ap-

pears to have resulted from a change in the balance of trace elements in the body. Roughage in the diet has been linked with an absence of cancer of the colon. Vitamin A appears capable of preventing lung cancer. And now moderate caloric restriction can prevent breast cancer, at least in laboratory animals, and vitamin C can extend the lives of terminal cancer patients." ("How Dietary Factors Combat Cancer," *Science News* 114 (November 13, 1976) p. 310-311.)

87 *Chinese distinction between food herbs and medicinal herbs*: I'm indebted for this explanation to Dr. Tei-Fu Chen, who holds an herbal pharmacy degree from Taiwan, and served as a physician in the Taiwanese Air Force. Dr. Chen actually describes three categories of herbs, and give other means of distinguishing them as well. I've oversimplified, feeling that my point didn't warrant a more complex explanation.

88 *Homeopathy*: For a comprehensive discussion of homeopathy, see Coulter, H. *Divided Legacy: A History of the Schism in Medical Thought*. Richmond, CA: North Atlantic Books, 1973, vol. 3.

89 *Homeopathy research*: For a comprehensive summary of scientific research on the homeopathic principle, see Coulter, H.L. *Homeopathic Science and Modern Medicine*. Richmond, CA: North Atlantic Books, 1981. • *Homeopathy and hay fever*: Reilly, D.T. et al. "Is Homoeopathy a Placebo Response? Controlled Trial of Homoeopathic Potency, with Pollen in Hayfever as Model." *Lancet* 8512 (November 29, 1986) p. 881-816. • *Homeopathy and arthritis*: Gibson, R.G. et al. "Homoeopathic Therapy in Rheumatoid Arthritis: Evaluation by Double-blind Clinical Therapeutic Trial." *British Medical Journal* 287 (July 30, 1983) p. 337-339. • *Homeopathy and colds*: Gassinger, C. A. et al. "A Controlled Clinical Trial for Testing the Efficacy of the Homeopathic Drug Eupatorium Perfoliatum D2 in the Treatment of Common Cold." *Arzneimittelforsch* 31 (1981) p. 732-736. • *Ar-*

tificial viruses: Bennett, D. W. "Drugs that Fight Cancer . . . naturally." *Science News* 128 (July 27, 1985) p. 58-61.

90 "less than heartening" and "at least you've tested": Both quotes taken from the Bennett reference cited directly above, p. 61.

Chapter 11
The Power of Personal Choice

Page

91 *"wise enough to choose"*: Jarvis, W.T. "Chiropractic: A Challenge for Health Education." *The Journal of School Health* 44 (April 1974) p. 213.

92 *Education*: Cassileth B. et al. "Contemporary Unorthodox Treatments in Cancer Medicine." *Annals of Internal Medicine* 101 (July 1984) p. 105-112. Another study showed that use of vitamin supplements rises directly with education. See Block, G. Et al. "Vitamin Supplement Use by Demographic Characteristics." *American Journal of Epidemiology* 127 (February, 1988) p. 297-309.

93 *Victims*: Taken form *The Professional's Guide to Health and Nutrition Fraud*. San Francisco: California Medical Association, (undated), p. 13-14. • *Norris quote*: Friend, T. "Cancer Fraud Lures Thousands." *USA Today* (March 17, 1988) p. 1D.

98 *Placebo responders*: "Who Responds Best to Placebos?" *Science News* 114 (January 24, 1976) p. 182. • *Greenhouse:* From an undated newsletter published by Arlo Richardson, Utah State Climatologist, Utah State University, Logan, Utah. • *Astronauts*: See "Osteoporosis and Activity." *Lancet* 8338 (June 18, 1983) p. 1365-1366. • *Normal adults*: Konner, M. *The Tangled Wing: Biological Constraints on the Human Spirit*. New York: Holt, Rinehart and Winston, 1982, p. 259

Chapter 12
Restrictive Health Laws are Not the Answer

Page

102 *FDA "drug" definition*: *The Professional's Guide to Health & Nutrition Fraud*. San Francisco: California Medical Association, (no date), p. 4.

103 *"built into the legislation": ACSH* [American Council on Science and Health] *News & Views* (November/December 1987) p. 13.

104 *Lysenko*: Broad, W. and Wade, N. *Betrayers of the Truth: Fraud and Deceit in the Halls of Science*. New York: Simon & Schuster, Inc., 1982, p. 186-192.

Chapter 13
Let's Fight Fraud With Freedom

Page

107 *Medical fraud*: Engler, R.L. et al. "Misrepresentation and Responsibility in Medical Research." *The New England Journal of Medicine* 317 (November 26, 1987) p. 1383-1389.

110 *Rubik*: Tierney, J. "The perplexing life of Erno Rubik." *Discover* (March 1986) p. 81-88.

111 *Correction of a defect in the cell's ability to move in response to a chemical signal*: Gatner, E.M. et al. "An *in vitro* Assessment of Cellular and Humoral Immune Function in Pulmonary Tuberculosis: Correction of Defective Neutrophil Molility by Ascorbate, Levamisole, Metoprolol and Propranolol." *Clinical and Experimental Immunology* 40 (May 1980) p. 327-326.) • *Improved migration and phagocytosis*: Thomas, W.R. et al. "Vitamin C and Immunity: An Assessment of the Evidence." *Clinical and Experimental Immunology* 32 (May 1978) p. 370-379.)

112 *Increased responsiveness of T cells and enhancement of interferon*: Siegel, B.V. et al. "Vitamin C and the Immune Response." *Experientia* 33 (March 15, 1977) p. 393-395.) • *Amplified*

production of antibodies: Prinz, W. et al. "A Systematic Study of the Effect of Vitamin C Supplementation on the Humoral Immune Response in Ascorbate-dependent Mammals." *International Journal of Vitamin and Nutrition Research* 50 (1980) p. 294-300.) • *Protection against anaphylactic shock*: Feigen, G.A. et al. "Enhancement of Antibody Production and Protection Against Systemic Anaphylaxis by Large Doses of Vitamin C." *Research Communications In Chemical Pathology and Pharmacology* 38 (November 1982) p. 313-333.) • *Inhibition of carcinogens and enhanced encapsulation of tumors*: Cameron, E. "Vitamin C and Cancer." *Internationale Zeitschrift fur Vitamin- Und Ernahrungforschung. Beiheft* 23 (1982) p. 115-127.) Collagen is connective tissue, and studies show that vitamin C helps form it, whether to encapsulate tumors, or in its normal function as part of our musculo-skeletal structure. The drug thalidomide apparently causes a decrease in systemic vitamin C, which could interfere with collagen formation, and some researchers speculate that's how the drug caused deformed limbs in children born of mothers who took it. (See Vaisman, B.L. et al. "Decrease in the Ascorbic Acid Content of Guinea Pig Tissues Caused by Thalidomide." *Biulleten Eksperimentalnoi Biologii I Meditsinyu* 96 (July 1983) p. 27-29. • *Chinese herb study*: Sun, Y. et al. "Immune Restoration and/or Augmentation of Local Graft Versus Host Reaction by Traditional Chinese Medicinal Herbs." *Cancer* 52 (July 1, 1983) p. 70-73. • *LA Times article:* "Chinese Derive Cancer Treatments from Ancient Herbal Tonics, Common Plants." *The Los Angeles Times*, October 6, 1983, part I-B, p. 5.

113 *$70 million per product*: Bunch, B. (ed.) *The Science Almanac*. Garden City, NY: Anchor Books, 1984, p. 483.

114 *Canals*: Hathaway, B. "The Ancient Canal that Turned Uphill." *Science 82* (October 1982) p. 80-

81. • *Mounds*: "Frost-free Indian Gardens." *Science News* 115 (February 12, 1977) p. 108. • *U.S. News*: "New Snake Oil, Old Pitch," *U.S. News &World Report* (December 8, 1986) p. 68-70. The article condemns evening primrose oil as unproven, despite the fact that it's used in hospitals throughout Europe, and dozens of articles attesting to its safety and effectiveness appear in medical journals, including the prestigious *Lancet*.

Appendix
A List of Natural Healing Resources

See also Linde, S. and Carrow, D.J. (eds) *The Directory of Holistic Medicine and Alternate Health Care Services in the U.S.* Phoenix, Arizona: Health Plus Publishers, 1985.

Index